KNOWN UNKNOWNS

OF EVERYDAY RADIOLOGY PRACTICE

A Practical Radiology Handbook

Demystifying Common
Patient Questions and Issues

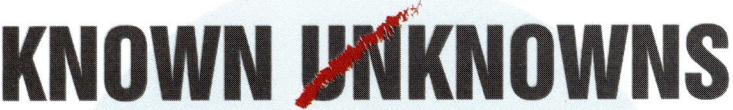

KNOWN UNKNOWNS

OF EVERYDAY RADIOLOGY PRACTICE

A Practical Radiology Handbook

Demystifying Common
Patient Questions and Issues

Bhavin Jankharia MD

Partner and Consultant, Picture This: Imaging and Beyond
Radiology Education Foundation
Mumbai

Akshay Baheti MD

Assistant Professor
Department of Radiodiagnosis
Tata Memorial Centre, Mumbai

Affiliate Instructor, Department of Body Imaging
University of Washington Medical Center
Seattle, USA

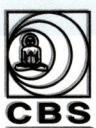

CBS

CBS Publishers & Distributors Pvt Ltd

New Delhi • Bengaluru • Chennai • Kochi • Kolkata • Lucknow • Mumbai

Hyderabad • Jharkhand • Nagpur • Patna • Pune • Uttarakhand

KNOWN UNKNOWNS
OF EVERYDAY RADIOLOGY PRACTICE
A Practical Radiology Handbook
Demystifying Common
Patient Questions and Issues

ISBN: 978-93-87085-87-9

Copyright © Authors and Publisher

Revised Reprint: 2019

Reprint: 2022

First Edition: 2018

Published by Satish Kumar Jain and produced by Varun Jain for

CBS Publishers & Distributors Pvt Ltd

4819/XI Prahlad Street, 24 Ansari Road, Daryaganj, New Delhi 110 002, India.

Ph: 011-23289259, 23266861, 23266867   Website: www.cbspd.com

Fax: 011-23243014   e-mail: delhi@cbspd.com; cbspubs@airtelmail.in

Corporate Office: 204 FIE, Industrial Area, Patparganj, Delhi 110 092

Ph: 011-49344934   Fax: 011-49344935   e-mail: publishing@cbspd.com; publicity@cbspd.com

Branches

- **Bengaluru:** Seema House 2975, 17th Cross, K.R. Road, Banasankari 2nd Stage, Bengaluru 560 070, Karnataka

  Ph: +91-80-26771678/79   Fax: +91-80-26771680   e-mail: bangalore@cbspd.com

- **Chennai:** 7, Subbaraya Street, Shenoy Nagar, Chennai 600 030, Tamil Nadu

  Ph: +91-44-26680620, 26681266   Fax: +91-44-42032115   e-mail: chennai@cbspd.com

- **Kochi:** 42/1325, 1326, Power House Road, Opp KSEB, Power House, Ernakulam 682 018, Kochi, Kerala, India

  Ph: +91-484-4059061-65   Fax: +91-484-4059065   e-mail: kochi@cbspd.com

- **Kolkata:** 147, Hind Ceramics Compound, 1st Floor, Nilgunj Road, Belghoria, Kolkata 700056, West Bengal

  Ph: +91-9096713055, 7798394118, 9836841399   e-mail: kolkata@cbspd.com

- **Lucknow:** Basement, Khushnuma Complex, 7-Meerabai Marg (Behind Jawahar Bhawan), Lucknow 226001, UP

  Ph: 0522-4000032   e-mail: tiwari.lucknow@cbspd.com

- **Mumbai:** PWD Shed. Gala no. 25/26, Ramchandra Bhatt Marg, Next to JJ Hospital Gate no. 2, Opp. Union Bank of India, Noorbaug, Mumbai-400009, Maharashtra, India

  Ph: 022-66661880/89   e-mail: mumbai@cbspd.com

Representatives

• **Hyderabad**	0-9885175004	• **Jharkhand**	0-9811541605	• **Nagpur**	0-9421945513
• **Patna**	0-9334159340	• **Pune**	0-9623451994	• **Uttarakhand**	0-9716462459

Printed at Goyal Offset Works Pvt. Ltd., Sonipat, Haryana, India

To

Our families who have stood with us through thick
and thin, and without whom this book would have been completed
6 months back!'

Bhavin and Akshay

To

My guru, philosopher and guide,
Dr Ravi Ramakantan, for teaching me not just
to make a diagnosis, but to make a difference.'

Akshay

Contributors

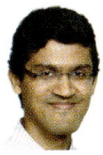

Akshay Baheti MD
Assistant Professor, Department of Radiodiagnosis, Tata Memorial Centre, Mumbai;
Affiliate Instructor, Department of Body Imaging, University of Washington, Medical Center, Seattle, USA.

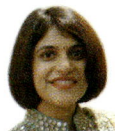

Aparna Katdare DMRD, DNB
Ex-Consultant Radiologist, Jankharia Imaging Centre, Mumbai

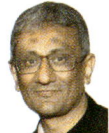

Bhavin Jankharia MD
Partner and Consultant, Picture this: Imaging and Beyond; Radiology Education Foundation, Mumbai

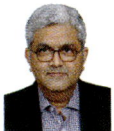

Milind Gune MD, DMRD, DMRE, FICR
Consultant Radiologist, Ambarnath (Thane), Maharashtra; Vice-Chairman, Indian College of Radiology and Imaging

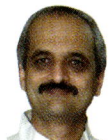

Samir Gandhi DNB
Consultant Radiologist and Proprietor, Gandhi Diagnostic Center, Mumbai; Treasurer, Maharashtra State Branch, Indian Radiological and Imaging Association; Secretary, Mumbai Chapter of Maharashtra State Chapter of IRIA; Ex-Lecturer, Seth GS Medical College and Lokmanya Tilak Medical College, Mumbai

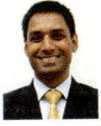

Sharad Maheshwari MD
Consultant Radiologist, Kokilaben Dhirubhai Ambani Hospital and Medical Research Institute, Mumbai

Foreword

"The questions you asked—the answers they never gave" is the phrase that comes to me as I write this Foreword to this small little piece of artwork.

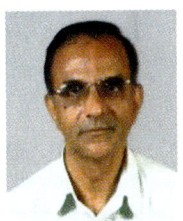

This book by Bhavin and Akshay changes all that—*now* you have all the answers!

The 11 chapters thoughtfully covered in this book are a gold mine of authoritative, referenced and easy to read and follow walkthrough through the landmines of everyday practice of radiology.

From information on the occasional encounter with the Atomic Energy Regulatory Board to the daily problem of administration of contrast, and everything in between that a radiologist will face in day-to-day practice; all of this is fully and clearly addressed in this book in such a way that rather than bumbling through answers which are half-truths, the radiologist can follow the path of the current state-of-the-art in the practice of radiology for the problem in question. For example, the chapter on Radiation Safety bursts the balloon of many myths that radiologists have on what is safe and what is not—a simple reading of this chapter will add great clarity to your practice and directly benefit patient care.

I particularly appreciate the chapter on Patient Rights and 'Un-rights' as this is a topic that is close to my heart; as clinical radiologists we ought to always look at ourselves as caregivers rather than the image-readers.

There is even a chapter on the fine art of performing a biopsy by image guidance. As you read through this chapter, you will realise that this is based on the vast experience of dealing with hundreds of biopsies and I feel this is a compulsory read for any radiologist who sticks in a needle into a patient under any image guidance.

And then, there is a chapter on what is wrong and right as far as handling radiology reports goes. I am sure every radiologist will learn something new by reading this chapter. This chapter is particularly important as the issues raised here are fraught with medicolegal consequences.

The authors have sought the help of other experts for some chapters and this adds authority and authenticity to the concerned information.

Even as I find it difficult not to mention more about the various chapters in this book, I do not wish this Foreword to be a summary of this book.

All that I want to say is: Buy this book for yourself— read it from skin to skin—even if it be a two-hour flight and you will be a much wiser radiologist and be able to spend a restful night's sleep as far as patient care and your practice are concerned.

The pages and the chapter headings are tastefully crafted, pleasing to the eye, as if, inviting you to read.

The only criticism of this book that I have is: "Why did not Bhavin and Akshay write this book earlier!"

If I sound extravagant in the praise of this book, I mean to be.

Ravi Ramakantan
Mumbai

A book like this is long overdue. Ever since we have worked with residents, both pre-DNB and post-MD and DNB, I have observed an utter lack of understanding of radiation and contrast media related issues among them.

This makes no sense.

When a patient asks a question, "What is my radiation risk", the patient and relatives expect that the answer will be given without fumbling, without beating around the bush and with the belief that these issues are an integral part of our core radiology curriculum.

The vast majority of radiologists, however, struggle with answers to such questions simply because they are rarely discussed in their departments or private clinics and the practices followed at most institutions are often incorrect and wrong.

Ever since the article by Brenner and Hall in the AJR in 2001, the whole issue of radiation risk has snowballed to unrecognizable proportions, to the extent that the equipment manufacturers have sunk billions of dollars developing technologies to reduce radiation dosage. A whole generation of radiologists and physicians and surgeons has grown up to believe intuitively that radiation is harmful. At a recent conference in Colombo, Sri Lanka, the interventional radiologist speaking about image-guided intervention in the chest was apologetic each time he spoke about CT-guided intervention, prefacing each case with the fact that radiation would be harmful to the patient, but because there was no choice, he had to do the procedure. This is insane and ridiculous.

The lay press has also not helped and keeps blowing out of proportion any article that talks about estimated radiation risk from computer simulations and calculations, a fact that stays in the minds of patients, adding to the mythology around this subject.

Similarly, when a patient presents with raised serum creatinine levels, many radiologists have no clue what to do, or work with some archaic system of beliefs that is completely out of sync with the current state of knowledge. Many hospitals and institutions are to blame, as the vast majority have no specific SOPs in place to address these issues, leading to consultants and residents taking decisions based on their "personal" experience or beliefs.

The same thing happens with pregnancy-related issues, where emotions rule rather than data and objectivity when making decisions. Obstetricians are clueless as well and often add to the misinformation that the patient is bombarded with. I still remember a lady who was pregnant with her third child and had undergone a chest radiograph in her 8th week of pregnancy. Her obstetrician sent her to me for counselling. I told her there was no risk to the fetus and she should continue the pregnancy. When she went back to her obstetrician, he told her he agreed with me, but if she were his wife, he would not continue the pregnancy. She terminated. What utter rubbish!!

Dr Akshay Baheti, my co-author, has recently returned from a 3-year stint in the US and is equally passionate about these subjects. We joined hands and started a course called RadPract, which is a one-day seminar that deals with the issues discussed in the book. We have had 3 meetings in 2017, with at least 3 more planned in 2018.

Realizing that we cannot reach everyone with these focused 20–30 members seminars, we decided to publish this book in an attempt to simplify issues related to the everyday practice of radiology … based on data, the experience of knowledge leaders, SOPs issued by international bodies, and the latest reviews on these subjects.

We have also added subjects related to consent during intervention and patient rights as well as the prickly issue of consent/information sheet prior to contrast media injections.

This book can pretty much be read in an hour or so, but more importantly can serve as a repository for information when faced with a sticky case or situation. We are extremely excited with this effort of ours, since no such book is currently available in India and for that matter, most parts of the world.

Bhavin Jankharia
November 2017

Contents

Chapter 1

Radiation and Patient Safety: Current Status

Bhavin Jankharia, Akshay Baheti

Clinical Scenarios

1. A 29-year-old man with past history of seminoma has had 4 prior CTs and comes for his 5th (surveillance) CT. He asks whether the risk of cancer is more on this 5th CT compared to the previous ones. What would be your response?
2. A 4-year-old boy comes for a CT abdomen for suspected neuroblastoma. How would you quantify his risk of developing cancer due to CT radiation? Is it higher than that of a 29-year-old man coming for a CT abdomen?
3. A 14-week by gestation pregnant patient with trauma needs an urgent CT study for further evaluation. She asks about the risk of fetal harm. What should be your answer?

INTRODUCTION

The potential cancer risk, if any, following low-dose radiation (as in diagnostic radiology procedures) is always a source of disquiet and hesitation in the minds of many radiologists, referring physicians, and patients alike. Unfortunately, over half a century of research in this field has not provided a definitive answer to this debate.[1] We provide a brief overview to the different theories of radiation-risk, and why we believe that based on current evidence, there is no reason to be worried about the radiation risk to patients in diagnostic radiology procedures, or to factor this into the decision-making process while deciding on performing a radiology investigation.

Linear No-threshold Model

Most of the data on radiation risk comes from the Japanese atomic bomb survivor cohort. Unfortunately, given that the survivors were exposed to a high level of radiation, the radiation risks for low-dose radiation exposure (<100 mGy) remain indeterminate and have been extrapolated from this data.[1, 2]

The model for assessing radiation risk currently endorsed by various international bodies including the National Council on Radiation Protection (NCRP) and Measurements, the International Council on Radiation Protection (ICRP), and the United Nations Scientific Committee on the Effects of Atomic Radiation is the linear no-threshold (LNT) model.[1] Simply put, this model directly extrapolates what happens at high radiation doses to low radiation doses. It states that the radiation-induced cancer risk is uniform across all doses, with no lower threshold below which the risk is negligible. In other words, the risk from a dose of 1 mGy is a thousand times less than the risk from a dose of a 1000 mGy; but is still a non-zero risk.[1, 2] Some authors have used this to throw in the arena several figures for excess cancers caused by diagnostic radiation exposure, even though the regulatory authorities have advised against such calculations.[3, 4] One group even projected up to 29,000 excess cancers caused by CT scans obtained in the US in 2007, an outrageous figure; while another projected 500 additional cancers per 10 mGy radiation exposure per million.[1, 5] Such misleading calculations and the adverse media publicity that they have received have led to the development of 'radiophobia' amongst physicians and patients alike.

In fact, subsequent to the Fukushima incident, the ICRP task force stated that "Following exposure to low radiation doses below about 100 mSv an increase of cancer has not been convincingly or consistently observed in epidemiological or experimental studies and will probably never be observed because of overwhelming statistical and biasing factors. In sum, theoretical cancer deaths after low-dose radiation exposure situations are obtained by inappropriate calculations based on the LNT model and misuse of the collective dose concept. Any effects—if they occur at all—will be so small that they would fall within the 'noise' (scatter) of the 'spontaneous' cancer of unexposed people".[6] The 2005 French Academy of Sciences Report also stated that there is no evidence for harm at radiation exposure <100 mGy and questioned the validity of using the LNT model at that level.[7]

The 'Hormetic' Model

The main problem with the linear no-threshold model is that it does not take into account the fact that the body does respond to radiation-induced cell level changes by various defense mechanisms such as DNA repair and apoptosis. For example, the spontaneous rate of mutations in the human body on an average is approximately 200,000 mutations per cell per day, which are taken care of by our defense mechanisms in almost all cases.[8] A CT study would on an average add about 10–100 more such mutations per cell; a miniscule figure.[2, 8] Epidemiological evidence, in fact, also suggests that low dose radiation exposure may actually lead to a *decreased* cancer incidence, indicating possible radiation 'hormesis'.[9] Hormesis is a toxicology term referring to a biphasic dose response to an agent characterized by a beneficial effect at a low dose and a harmful effect at a higher dose (exemplified by the quote 'one man's medicine is another man's poison'). This is probably due to the beneficial effects from activation of the body's immune response.

A third 'threshold' model suggests that there is a threshold below which radiation does not lead to increased cancer risk. If the radiation exposure is higher than this threshold, then there is a possible risk of excess cancer. Figure 1.1 explains these radiation risk models well.

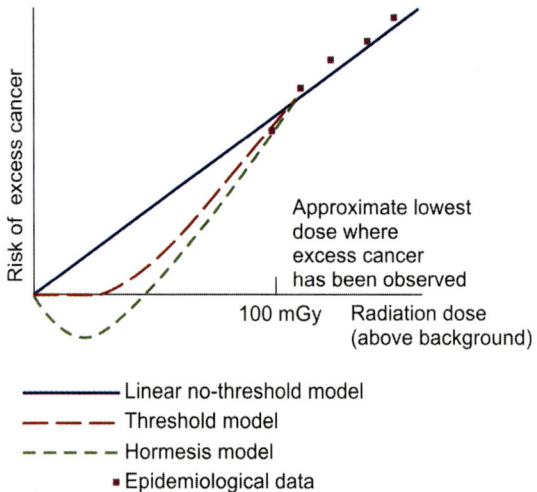

Fig. 1.1: Models for risk of excess cancer from exposure to low dose of ionizing radiation (adapted from the Canadian Nuclear Safety Commission website)

(http://nuclearsafety.gc.ca/eng/resources/health/linear-non-threshold-model/index.cfm; accessed on 28.07.17). The black data points at around 100 mGy and above are taken from epidemiological studies (including studies on radon in homes, nuclear energy workers, medical exposures and the atomic bomb survivors) by the Commission.

Estimated Radiation Doses to Adults from Common Imaging Examinations

Table 1.1 gives the estimated radiation doses which a typical adult would receive after undergoing certain common imaging studies as per ACR. It is quite clear that the radiation exposure even after a PET/CT is far less than what would be a cause of concern.

Please note that while these are published figures by ACR, as per institutional unpublished data (Tata Memorial Hospital, Mumbai), single-phase routine CECT abdomen and pelvis on a 16-slice scanner (Siemens Somatom) using automatic exposure control with a collimation of 1.2 mm and 0.6 mm can lead to an average radiation dose of approximately 13 mGy and 14.5 mGy respectively. Thus, every institute should try to evaluate their own data regarding radiation exposure.

Table 1.1: Estimated radiation doses to adults from common imaging examinations (ACR data)

Examination	Dose (mGy)
CT abdomen and pelvis	10
CT chest	7
CT head	2
Cardiac CT	12
Chest X-ray	0.1
PET/CT	25

'Radiophobia': Demolishing Some Myths

The few sensational articles giving large estimates of radiation-induced carcinogenesis have led to the development of 'radiophobia' in the minds of patients and physicians, and indeed radiologists as well. Public campaigns like the 'Image Gently' campaign have developed amongst the radiology community as a reactionary measure to tackle this issue. While there is no doubt that excess radiation exposure should be avoided (appropriate scans need to be performed depending on the indication of the study), the fallout of this radiophobia has been that many studies are suboptimal due to utilization of low dose algorithms. Indeed, as many as 1 in 20 pediatric CTs may not be of adequate diagnostic quality in USA due to excessive focus on limiting radiation exposure.[2] This completely removes the 'reasonably' component from the ALARA (as low as reasonably achievable) principle. Thus, rather than *decreasing* radiation exposure, the focus ought to be on *optimizing* radiation exposure.[10]

Importantly, many amongst the medical and patient community are also hesitant in requesting indicated CTs in patients with prior history of radiation exposure.[11] This despite the fact that potential carcinogenesis is a stochastic effect, which means that prior radiation exposure will have no bearing on the risk of developing cancer due to a future CT. In other words, a 35-year-old male with history of seminoma and 5 prior CT abdomen studies will have the same theoretical radiation risk of developing cancer due to his 6th CT study as another 35-year-old male undergoing a CT abdomen for the first time for suspected pancreatitis. It is important to stop factoring prior CTs into the decision-making process, and educate our medical colleagues about the same.

Pediatric patients have been purported to be at a higher lifetime risk of developing radiation-associated cancer as they are assumed to be more radiosensitive (besides having a longer lifespan), leading to a special focus on them.[10] A few large epidemiological studies have famously observed a correlation between pediatric CTs and subsequent development of cancer.[12,13] However, these results have been questioned even by the NCRP chairman, and the association is likely due to reverse causation (patients who developed cancers were more likely to have had a CT scan due to the presence of predisposing syndromes such as myelodysplasia).[14] More recent studies in the pediatric patient population which adjusted for such factors, in fact, did not demonstrate any significant excess cancer risk.[15,16] A similar study in patients (both pediatric and adult population) who had undergone a CT head did not find an increased risk in the development of a meningioma in them, after excluding patients who already had a meningioma at the time of the first CT and those who had received radiation therapy.[17] Thus, it would be more prudent to again focus on radiation optimization rather than radiation reduction in pediatric patients.

A new theory published recently is about the increased risk of radiation caused by the iodinated contrast media itself within vessels and tissues when it interacts with the X-rays,[18] a theory that has been successfully challenged and debunked in the same issue of the journal.[19]

Conclusion

In conclusion, based on the current literature, the radiation risks for carcinogenesis are certainly no cause for concern, and are most likely non-existent. In fact, certain data suggests that low dose radiation may have a beneficial effect (hormesis). Incidentally, the background annual radiation exposure of patients living in certain parts of Kerala is as high as 70 mGy, without increased cancer incidence.[8] Another similar reassuring fact is that even in pregnant women, ICRP states that radiation exposure up to 50 mGy does not have any deleterious deterministic effect on the baby (to be discussed in more detail in Chapter 3).[20] ICRP also states that for exposures between 50 and 100 mGy, 'potential effects are scientifically uncertain and probably too subtle to be clinically detectable'.[20] Compare this with the average radiation exposure of a single phase CT abdomen and pelvis study, which is approximately 10–15 mGy.[21]

It is thus obvious that the risk of radiation oncogenesis is probably zero, and in any case grossly exaggerated. The real risk of delayed or incorrect diagnosis due to not ordering an indicated CT or substituting it with a USG is much more than this hypothetical risk. Clinical decision-making should certainly not be influenced to the slightest bit by the 'risk' of diagnostic radiation-associated cancer development, nor by previous history of radiation exposure.

AT A GLANCE

- The reliance on the linear no-threshold model has led to undue scare-mongering about the "dangers" of diagnostic imaging related radiation exposure.
- Single dose exposures of less than 100 mGy are not associated with any evidence of increased risk of carcinogenesis.
- Cumulative exposure does not lead to increased risk, since each exposure is its own stochastic event.
- Current epidemiological data demonstrates that children are not more radiosensitive than adults, and hence the same rules apply to them.
- Similarly, low-dose diagnostic radiation is safe in pregnancy across all stages of pregnancy.

Clinical Scenarios

Q1. *A 29-year-old man with past history of seminoma has had 4 prior CTs and comes for his 5th (surveillance) CT. He asks whether the risk of cancer is more on this 5th CT compared to the previous ones. What would be your response?*

Ans: Radiation being a scholastic effect, the risk of every CT is individual and not cumulative. There is no current data to demonstrate any increased risk of cancer at the dose he will receive from the CT. Nevertheless, any theoretical risk from this 5th CT is going to be the same as the risk in each of the prior 4 CTs.

Q2. *A 4-year-old boy comes for a CT abdomen for suspected neuroblastoma. How would you quantify his risk of developing cancer due to CT radiation? Is it higher than that of a 29-year-old man coming for a CT abdomen?*

Ans: There is no current data to demonstrate any increased risk of cancer at the dose the boy will receive from the CT. Nevertheless, any theoretical risk from the CT will be similar to that of a 29-year-old man.

Q3. *A 14-week by gestation pregnant patient with trauma needs an urgent CT abdomen and pelvis study for further evaluation. She asks about the risk of fetal harm. What should be your answer?*

Ans: As per the ICRP guidelines, fetal radiation up to 50 mGy causes no fetal harm at any gestational age (details in Chapter 3). Since a single phase CT will cause only about 10–15 mGy of exposure, the baby should not have any risk from the study. Not performing the CT will, on the other hand, lead to a definite risk of missing a serious internal injury, which does have a higher risk of increased maternal and fetal morbidity and mortality.

Suggested Further Reading

1. Siegel JA, Pennington CW, Sacks B. Subjecting Radiologic Imaging to the Linear No-Threshold Hypothesis: A Non Sequitur of Non-Trivial Proportion. J Nucl Med 2017;58:1–6.

2. Siegel JA, Sacks B, Pennington CW, Welsh JS. Dose Optimization to Minimize Radiation Risk for Children Undergoing CT and Nuclear Medicine Imaging Is Misguided and Detrimental. J Nucl Med 2017;58:865–68.

3. Siegel JA, Welsh JS. Does Imaging Technology Cause Cancer? Debunking the Linear No-Threshold Model of Radiation Carcinogenesis. Technol Cancer Res Treat 2016;15:249–56.

4. Weber W, Zanzonico P. The Controversial Linear No-Threshold Model. J Nucl Med 2017;58:7–8.

REFERENCES

1. Weber W, Zanzonico P. The Controversial Linear No-Threshold Model. J Nucl Med 2017;58:7–8.

2. Siegel JA, Pennington CW, Sacks B. Subjecting Radiologic Imaging to the Linear No-Threshold Hypothesis: A Non Sequitur of Non-Trivial Proportion. J Nucl Med 2017;58:1–6.

3. Brenner D, Elliston C, Hall E, Berdon W. Estimated risks of radiation-induced fatal cancer from pediatric CT. AJR Am J Roentgenol 2001;176:289–96.

4. Brenner DJ, Hall EJ. Computed tomography—an increasing source of radiation exposure. N Engl J Med 2007;357:2277–84.

5. Berrington de Gonzalez A, Mahesh M, Kim KP, et al. Projected cancer risks from computed tomographic scans performed in the United States in 2007. Arch Intern Med 2009;169:2071–7.

6. Gonzalez AJ, Akashi M, Boice JD, Jr., et al. Radiological protection issues arising during and after the Fukushima nuclear reactor accident. J Radiol Prot 2013;33:497–571.

7. Tubiana M. Dose-effect relationship and estimation of the carcinogenic effects of low doses of ionizing radiation: the joint report of the Academie des Sciences (Paris) and of the Academie Nationale de Medecine. Int J Radiat Oncol Biol Phys 2005;63:317–9.

8. Siegel JA, Welsh JS. Does Imaging Technology Cause Cancer? Debunking the Linear No-Threshold Model of Radiation Carcinogenesis. Technol Cancer Res Treat 2016;15:249–56.

9. Sasaki MS, Tachibana A, Takeda S. Cancer risk at low doses of ionizing radiation: artificial neural networks inference from atomic bomb survivors. J Radiat Res 2014;55:391–406.

10. Siegel JA, Sacks B, Pennington CW, Welsh JS. Dose Optimization to Minimize Radiation Risk for Children Undergoing CT and

Nuclear Medicine Imaging Is Misguided and Detrimental. J Nucl Med 2017;58:865–68.

11. Pandharipande PV, Eisenberg JD, Avery LL, et al. Journal club: How radiation exposure histories influence physician imaging decisions: a multicenter radiologist survey study. AJR Am J Roentgenol 2013;200:1275–83.

12. Mathews JD, Forsythe AV, Brady Z, et al. Cancer risk in 680,000 people exposed to computed tomography scans in childhood or adolescence: data linkage study of 11 million Australians. BMJ 2013;346:f2360

13. Pearce MS, Salotti JA, Little MP, et al. Radiation exposure from CT scans in childhood and subsequent risk of leukaemia and brain tumours: a retrospective cohort study. Lancet 2012;380: 499–505.

14. Boice JD, Jr. Radiation epidemiology and recent paediatric computed tomography studies. Ann ICRP 2015;44:236–48.

15. Journy N, Rehel JL, Ducou Le Pointe H, et al. Are the studies on cancer risk from CT scans biased by indication? Elements of answer from a large-scale cohort study in France. Br J Cancer 2015;112:185–93.

16. Krille L, Dreger S, Schindel R, et al. Risk of cancer incidence before the age of 15 years after exposure to ionising radiation from computed tomography: results from a German cohort study. Radiat Environ Biophys 2015;54:1–12.

17. Nordenskjold AC, Bujila R, Aspelin P, Flodmark O, Kaijser M. Risk of Meningioma after CT of the Head. Radiology 2017:1614–33.

18. Sahbaee P, Abadi E, Segars WP, Marin D, Nelson RC, Samei E. The Effect of Contrast Material on Radiation Dose at CT: Part II. A Systematic Evaluation across 58 Patient Models. Radiology 2017;283:749–57.

19. Boone JM, Hernandez AM. The Effect of Iodine-based Contrast Material on Radiation Dose at CT: It's Complicated. Radiology 2017;283:624–27.

20. Wang PI, Chong ST, Kielar AZ, et al. Imaging of pregnant and lactating patients: part 1, evidence-based review and recommendations. AJR Am J Roentgenol 2012;198:778–84.

21. American College of Radiology. Radiation Dose to Adults from Common Imaging Examinations. https://www.acr.org/~/media/ACR/Documents/PDF/QualitySafety/Radiation-Safety/Dose-Reference-Card.pdf. Accessed on 28.6.17.

Chapter 2

Contrast Media: Current Guidelines for Iodinated and Gadolinium-based Contrast Administration

Akshay Baheti, Sharad Maheshwari

Clinical Scenarios

1. A patient with chronic kidney disease (CKD) is referred for an indicated CECT of the abdomen with a serum creatinine of 1.9 mg/dl (eGFR of 33). Would you perform the CECT?
2. A patient with CKD is referred for an indicated CT pulmonary angiogram (CTPA) with a serum creatinine of 2.5 mg/dl (eGFR of 23). Would you perform the CTPA?
3. A CKD patient with scheduled dialysis tomorrow needs an urgent CTPA; the dialysis cannot be preponed. Should you do it now or wait till tomorrow?
4. A patient with diabetes and serum creatinine of 2.1 (eGFR of 28) comes for an elective CECT of the abdomen. He tells you he is on metformin and just took the dose in the morning before coming for the CT. Should you perform the CT or delay it?
5. A CKD patient on dialysis with suspected brain tumor needs a CE-MRI. Would you do it or not? If yes, which contrast would you use?
6. A CKD patient with scheduled dialysis tomorrow needs an indicated CE-MRI; the dialysis cannot be preponed. Should you do it now or wait till tomorrow?

A. IODINATED CONTRAST MEDIA

Points to Note

- IV contrast-induced nephropathy, henceforth referred to as post-contrast acute kidney injury (AKI), is defined as an increase in serum creatinine ≥ 0.5 mg/dl or $\geq 25\%$ from baseline within 1–3 days after administration of IV contrast, in the absence of other risk factors. Historically, the concept of post-contrast AKI developed in the 1950s and 60s during the pre-CT days of high-osmolar contrast media, based mainly on intra-arterial angiography literature. This should not be extrapolated to intravenous studies using low-osmolar contrast media.

- A few recent landmark studies by McDonald et al and Davenport et al have demonstrated that the risk of post-contrast AKI has been grossly exaggerated, and contrast is possibly not nephrotoxic at all, or at worst a weak independent nephrotoxic agent. A recent meta-analysis by Aycock et al of over 1 lakh patients also concluded that acute kidney injury, need for renal replacement therapy, and all-cause mortality were not significantly different in patients receiving IV contrast compared to patients who underwent a non-contrast CT.

- Based on current literature, post-contrast AKI is at best a rare entity. As per ACR guidelines, if a cut-off needs to be set, eGFR (estimated glomerular filtration rate) <30 ml/min/1.73 m^2 is the best cut-off. Based on the current evidence and guidelines, we have suggested a policy for IV contrast administration in patients with renal dysfunction (Table 2.1).

- eGFR is a more accurate indicator of renal function compared to serum creatinine. eGFR can be easily calculated online using the MDRD formula. Many free apps are also available to download which can calculate eGFR using the MDRD equation. Other fomulae (such as Cockcroft-Gault) should not be used as all current literature on post-contrast AKI is based on eGFR values calculated using the MDRD formula.

- There is no definite evidence to prove that IV contrast dose and rate of injection have any association with the development of post-contrast AKI.

- Suspected risk factors for post-contrast AKI include age >60 years, renal disease (dialysis, renal cancer, renal transplant, single kidney, renal surgery), diabetes, hypertension, and patient on nephrotoxic drugs. Also, eliciting history of metformin use is important.

- Traditionally, repeat studies using contrast have been avoided within 24 hours of each other. However, there is no evidence to prove its utility in preventing post-contrast AKI, and the ACR does not endorse this practice. There is no need to repeat

Table 2.1: Suggested cut-offs for IV contrast administration in patients with renal dysfunction	
eGFR <45 ml/min/1.73 m^2	Administer full dose contrast
eGFR 30–44 ml/min/1.73 m^2	Administer full dose contrast. May give prophylactic hydration (see below)
eGFR <30 ml/min/1.73 m^2, or patients with acute renal failure and any eGFR value	Direct consultation with referring physician and administration of contrast on a case-by-case basis; prefer to avoid giving contrast if alternatives exist, but keep the threshold to give contrast low if there is clinical benefit. Prophylactic hydration needed for all.
Patients on dialysis	See ahead

serum creatinine in between two such studies either (as creatinine changes lag behind worsening renal function).

PROPHYLACTIC MEASURES TO PREVENT POST-CONTRAST AKI

- Hydrating the patient prior to administering contrast is the standard of care. IV hydration is said to be probably superior to oral hydration as per the ACR contrast guidelines, although this too may be relaxed for patients with eGFR >30 ml/min/1.73 m^2 (discussed below).
- For oral hydration, advise intake of at least 500 cc of water over 2 hours before and another 500 cc over 2 hours after the study.
- For IV hydration, use isotonic fluids (NS or Ringer lactate). Give 0.9% NS 1 ml/kg/hour for 6–12 hours before and 6–12 hours after the procedure for inpatients. Give 0.9% NS 3 ml/kg/hour for 1 hour before and 1–1.5 ml/kg/hour for 4–6 hours (totally 6 ml/kg cumulative) after the procedure for outpatients if they cannot drink orally.
- Evidence for using sodium bicarbonate is weak, but is an option for the clinician.
- There is no conclusive evidence that iso-osmolar contrast (Visipaque) is less nephrotoxic than low-osmolar contrast

(Omipaque/Ultravist). Visipaque may be preferred if there is volume overload/patient on dialysis.

- Evidence for a reno-protective role of N-acetylcysteine (NAC) is weak, and it is not necessary to give NAC for prophylaxis. NAC is often administered nevertheless due to it being relatively inexpensive and non-toxic, and because the referring clinicians are more comfortable with this approach. It may be given in four doses of 600 mg each, two prior (24 and 12 hours) and two after (12 and 24 hours) the contrast administration.

- A recent prospective randomized controlled phase III study published in Lancet in 2017 by Nijssen et al compared prophylactic IV hydration to no hydration in patients with eGFR between 30 and 59 ml/min/1.73 m^2, and found no hydration to be non-inferior and more cost-effective. In other words, hydration probably does not have any prophylactic role in preventing the development of nephropathy in patients with eGFR between 30 and 59 ml/min/1.73 m^2. This finding makes intuitive sense given the recent studies demonstrating that contrast-induced nephropathy (CIN) does not probably exist in patients with eGFR ≥30 ml/min/1.73 m^2.

- Given this data, while the current guidelines do recommend hydration as the standard of care, it might be acceptable to relax this need in patients with eGFR 30–44 ml/min/1.73 m^2, particularly in urgent patients in whom it might not be safe to wait the extra hours for hydration, or in patients who have volume overload. However, do note that the current ESUR guidelines (as on 8.10.2017) recommend giving hydration in this set of patients.

Metformin

- Patients on metformin are not at a higher risk of post-contrast AKI. However, they are at a risk of developing lactic acidosis if they do develop post-contrast AKI.
- In patients with eGFR ≥30 ml/min/1.73 m^2, there is no need to discontinue metformin.

- In patients with eGFR <30 ml/min/1.73 m^2, discontinue metformin at the time of scan and restart after 48 hours after a renal function test has been performed.
- Metformin can be continued in patients receiving gadolinium.

Dialysis

- Hemodialysis has no proven role in preventing post-contrast AKI. While contrast administration should be avoided if reasonable alternatives exist, contrast should not be withheld if there is a genuine clinical need for it.
- In patients on routine dialysis, correlation of contrast administration with the timing of hemodialysis is not necessary.
- In particular, do not hesitate in giving contrast in anuric CKD patients on dialysis, as there is no substantial remaining renal function present in them anyway to harm.
- Continuous ambulatory peritoneal dialysis patients do not need a hemodialysis session after IV iodinated contrast.

B. GADOLINIUM-BASED CONTRAST MEDIA

- Based on their chemical structure, gadolinium-based contrast agents are classified as either linear agents or macrocyclic agents. Linear agents are further classified as ionic or non-ionic agents (Table 2.2).
- With regards to stability, macrocyclic agents are more stable than linear ionic agents, which in turn are more stable than linear non-ionic agents.

Table 2.2: Linear ionic and non-ionic agents		
Linear non-ionic	Linear ionic	Macrocyclic
Optimark	Magnevist	Dotarem
Omniscan	Multihance	Gadavist
Eovist	Prohance	

CONTRAST AGENTS TO USE AND TO AVOID IN PATIENTS WITH eGFR <30 ml/min/1.73 m²

- As per both ESUR and ACR guidelines, Optimark, Omniscan, and Magnevist (group I agents) have the highest risk of nephrogenic systemic fibrosis (NSF) and are contraindicated.
- Based on the current evidence and guidelines, we have suggested a policy for IV gadolinium contrast administration in patients with renal dysfunction (Table 2.3).
- **Prefer to use macrocyclic contrast agents as they have the lowest risk of NSF (ESUR guidelines).** Another alternative is to use Multihance (intermediate risk of NSF as per ESUR but safe as per ACR). Few, if any, unconfounded cases of NSF have been reported with these agents.
- Eovist is a new agent with not enough data available on its use vis-à-vis NSF; it is classified as intermediate risk by ESUR.
- As per ACR guidelines, eGFR between 30 and 40 ml/min/1.73 m² should be considered equivalent with that <30, as eGFR values can have mild daily variations. However, ESUR does not mention this additional cut-off. Nonetheless, it may be prudent to use a macrocyclic agent in this group of patients as well.

Table 2.3: Suggested cut-offs for contrast administration in patients with renal dysfunction*	
eGFR >30 ml/min/1.73 m²	Administer full dose contrast.
eGFR <30 ml/min/1.73 m², or patients with acute renal failure	Avoid contrast administration. Prefer non-contrast MRI or a CECT. Contrast (preferably macrocyclic agents: Dotarem, Gadavist or Prohance) may be administered if there is sufficient clinical concern and if no other option exists, and after a radiologist–physician discussion and informed patient consent.

Dialysis

- Role of dialysis in preventing NSF is uncertain; cases of NSF have been reported in patients on dialysis.
- Hemodialysis, however, remains the standard of care currently as per both ACR and ESUR guidelines. It should be performed immediately after MRI examination (MRI examination should be scheduled as per the dialysis appointment).
- Multiple sessions of dialysis have not been proven beyond doubt to be helpful, but may be performed as per the referring physician/nephrologist's requirements.
- Patients on continuous ambulatory peritoneal dialysis need to undergo hemodialysis as well.

The following is a suggested list of risk factors that warrants pre-administration eGFR calculation in individuals scheduled to receive a gadolinium injection as per ACR (Table 2.4).

1. Age >60 years
2. History of renal disease, including dialysis, renal transplant, history of renal surgery, history of renal cancer, or a single kidney

Table 2.4: When to get eGFR/serum creatinine testing for MRI in the general population (ACR guidelines)		
Previous eGFR value	*When was it obtained?*	*When should a new eGFR be obtained?*
None		<6 weeks
>60	>6 months	<6 weeks
	<6 months (stable)*	Not needed
	<6 months (unstable)**	<2 weeks
30–59		<2 weeks
<30		<1 week
Dialysis		Not needed

*Patient does not have any condition which may lead to acute deterioration of renal function.
**Patient has a known condition that may lead to acute deterioration of renal function (dehydration, fever, sepsis, heart failure, recent hospitalization, etc.)

3. Hypertension requiring medical therapy

4. Diabetes mellitus

GADOLINIUM DEPOSITION IN BRAIN

- Gadolinium can and does deposit in the brain (particularly dentate nucleus and globus pallidus) in patients with normal renal function. The risk is higher with linear contrast agents compared to macrocyclic agents.

- Macrocyclic agents (Dotarem, Prohance, and Gadovist) are safer to use in this regard as they cause less deposition as compared to the linear agents.

- The clinical significance of gadolinium deposition in the brain is uncertain. A large retrospective study by Welk et al (JAMA 2016) did not find any correlation between gadolinium administration and development of Parkinsonism. Another large study by McDonald et al (presented at RSNA 2017) reviewed the findings of an ongoing prospective cohort study (Mayo Clinic Study on Aging) and did not find any association between gadolinium administration and neurocognitive decline. The current consensus amongst all organizations is that there is no definite proof of clinically significant harm caused by gadolinium deposition.

- However, given that safer macrocyclic agents are available in the market, the European Medicines Agency has recommended suspension of marketing authorization of the linear agents (Optimark, Omniscan, and Magnevist) given the current data. This essentially means that linear agents have been banned in all European Union member states.

- Macrocyclic agents remain approved in the EU. Eovist and Multihance are approved for use solely as a hepatocyte-specific contrast agent (and not for other purposes), as there is no macrocyclic counterpart for this purpose. Intra-articular use of Magnevist is also approved given the low dose utilized.

- Japan has also recommended the use of linear agents to only when no macrocyclic alternatives exist.
- US-FDA, ACR and the Radiological Society of North America (RSNA) have disagreed, given that currently no clinically significant effect has been demonstrated due to gadolinium deposition. They state that they will continue to monitor the situation closely, but have decided against a ban on linear agents as of now. The International Society for Magnetic Resonance in Medicine also endorses this view. The US-FDA however has mandated to add a warning on potential gadolinium retention to GBCA labels.
- Given these diverse views, there is no medicolegal compulsion on avoiding the use of linear gadolinium contrast agents in India as of now. However, it might be prudent to prefer using macrocyclic agents in at least children, young adults, and potentially repeat users, if not in all patients.

AT A GLANCE

- eGFR (calculated using MDRD formula) is a more reliable measure of renal function compared to serum creatinine, and should be used to make decisions regarding contrast administration.
- Recent data suggests that it is safe to administer IV contrast in all patients with eGFR >30 ml/min/1.73 m^2 without causing any nephrotoxicity. Even in patients with eGFR <30 ml/min/1.73 m^2, contrast is at worst a weak independent risk factor for developing nephropathy.
- CIN is thus grossly over-estimated by both radiologists and clinicians. The risk of undergoing a non-diagnostic non-contrast CT is probably higher than the potential risk of developing CIN even in many patients with low eGFR. Hence, in patients with eGFR <30 ml/min/1.73 m^2, it is best to talk to the referring doctor about the indication of the study and decide on a case-by-case basis whether IV contrast should be administered.

- Prophylactic hydration is the standard of care for CIN prophylaxis, although its role remains equivocal. There is no conclusive evidence that using NAC or Visipaque prevents the development of nephropathy.
- Amongst gadolinium-based contrast media, macrocyclic agents are the most stable and safest to use in patients with risk of developing NSF (patients on dialysis, patients with eGFR <30 ml/min/1.73 m^2, or patients with acute renal failure) or in pregnant women. Magnevist, Optimark, and Omniscan are contra-indicated.
- Gadolinium deposits in brain in small amounts, even in individuals with normal renal function. No clinically significant side-effect has yet been proven due to this. Macrocyclics are again safer in this regard. Currently, the US-FDA continues to approve all agents for use, while the EU has suspended the use of most linear agents as described in the text.

Answers to Clinical Scenarios

Q1. *A patient with chronic kidney disease (CKD) is referred for an indicated contrast enhanced CT (CECT) of the abdomen with a creatinine of 1.9 mg/dL (eGFR of 33). Would you perform the CECT?*

Ans: Yes; give full dose contrast, with oral or IV hydration as prophylaxis.

Q2. *A patient with CKD is referred for an indicated CTPA with a creatinine of 2.5 mg/dL (eGFR of 23). Would you perform the CTPA?*

Ans: Personally talk to the referring physician and if it is truly indicated (elevated D-dimer in a breathless patient with normal lower limb Doppler), perform the study. Give full dose contrast, along with prophylactic hydration.

Q3. *A CKD patient with scheduled dialysis tomorrow needs an urgent CTPA; the dialysis cannot be preponed. Should you do it now or wait till tomorrow?*

Ans: It can be performed right away.

Q4. *A patient with diabetes and serum creatinine of 2.1 (eGFR of 28) comes for a routine CECT of the abdomen. He tells you he is on metformin and just took the dose in the morning before coming for the CT. Should you perform the CT or delay it?*

Ans: CT can be performed and the patient should be asked not to take metformin for the next 48 hours. A serum creatinine value should be repeated thereafter, and metformin may be restarted depending on the test results.

Q5. *A CKD patient on dialysis with suspected brain tumor needs a CE-MRI. Would you do it or not? If yes, which contrast would you use?*

Ans: Yes; CE-MRI should be performed using a macrocyclic agent.

Q6. *A CKD patient with scheduled dialysis tomorrow needs an indicated CE-MRI; the dialysis cannot be preponed. Should you do it now or wait till tomorrow?*

Ans: Preferably wait till tomorrow and perform the study as close to the hemodialysis session as possible.

Suggested Further Reading

1. Bettmann MA. Frequently Asked Questions: Iodinated Contrast Agents. Radiographics 2004; 24:S3–S10.
2. Davenport MS, Cohan RH, Ellis JH. Contrast media controversies in 2015: imaging patients with renal impairment or risk of contrast reaction. Am J Roentgenol 2015;204:1174–81.
3. Davenport MS, Cohan RH, Khalatbari S, Ellis JH. The Challenges in Assessing Contrast-Induced Nephropathy: Where Are We Now? Am J Roentgenol 2014; 202:784–789.
4. ESUR Contrast Media Guidelines version 8.1. Accessed from http://www.esur.org/guidelines/
5. Manual on Contrast Media v10.3. Accessed from https://www.acr.org/Quality-Safety/Resources/Contrast-Manual

BIBLIOGRAPHY

1. Aycock RD, Westafer LM, Boxen JL, Majlesi N, Schoenfeld EM, Bannuru RR. Acute Kidney Injury After Computed Tomography: A Meta-analysis. *Ann Emerg Med* 2017.

2. Davenport MS, Khalatbari S, Cohan RH, Dillman JR, Myles JD, Ellis JH. Contrast material-induced nephrotoxicity and intravenous low-osmolality iodinated contrast material: risk stratification by using estimated glomerular filtration rate. *Radiology* 2013;268:719–28.

3. ESUR Contrast Media Guidelines version 8.1. Accessed from http://www.esur.org/guidelines/on 28.7.17.

4. European Medicines Agency Press Release. Accessed from http://www.ema.europa.eu/ema/index.jsp?curl=pages/news_and_events/news/2017/03/news_detail_002708.jsp&mid=WC0b01ac058004d5c1 on 3.4.17.

5. Gulani V, Calamante F, Shellock FG, Kanal E, Reeder SB; on behalf of International Society for Magnetic Resonance in Medicine. Gadolinium deposition in the brain: summary of evidence and recommendations. *Lancet Neurol* 2017;16:564–70.

6. Kanda T, Ishii K, Kawaguchi H, Kitajima K, Takenaka D. High signal intensity in the dentate nucleus and globus pallidus on unenhanced T1-weighted MR images: relationship with increasing cumulative dose of a gadolinium-based contrast material. *Radiology* 2014;270:834–41.

7. Manual on Contrast Media v10.3. Accessed from https://www.acr.org/Quality-Safety/Reso-urces/Contrast-Manual on 28.7.17.

8. McDonald JS, McDonald RJ, Carter RE, Katzberg RW, Kallmes DF, Williamson EE. Risk of intravenous contrast material-mediated acute kidney injury: a propensity score-matched study stratified by baseline-estimated glomerular filtration rate. *Radiology* 2014;271:65–73.

9. Welk B, McArthur E, Morrow SA, MacDonald P, Hayward J, Leung A, et al. Association Between Gadolinium Contrast Exposure and the Risk of Parkinsonism. JAMA 2016;316:96-8.

10. McDonald RJ, McDonald JS, Therneau T, Eckel LJ, Kallmes DF, Carter R, et al. Assessment of the neurologic effects of intracranial gadolinium deposition using a large population based cohort. RSNA 2017.

11. Nijssen EC, Rennenberg RJ, Nelemans PJ, et al. Prophylactic hydration to protect renal function from intravascular iodinated contrast material in patients at high risk of contrast-induced nephropathy (AMACING): a prospective, randomized, phase 3, controlled, open-label, non-inferiority trial. Lancet 2017; 389: 1312–22.

12. Olchowy C, Cebulski K, Lasecki M, et al. The presence of the gadolinium-based contrast agent depositions in the brain and symptoms of gadolinium neurotoxicity—A systematic review. *PLoS One* 2017;12:e0171704.

Chapter 3

CT and MRI in Pregnancy: Current Status

Akshay Baheti, Aparna Katdare, Bhavin Jankharia

Clinical Scenarios

1. A 10-week pregnant lady with a single live fetus on a recent USG had a single-phase CT abdomen at 4 weeks. How high is the risk of the baby developing a malformation due to the CT? Should she abort or not?

2. A 14-week pregnant patient needs a CECT abdomen and pelvis. What should you be extremely worried about: Fetal radiation exposure, fetal renal toxicity, or fetal thyroid toxicity?

3. A 14-week pregnant patient needs an MRI pelvis for suspected AVN of hip. Your hospital has both a 1.5T MRI and a 3T MRI. Are both equally safe or would you prefer using one over the other?

4. A 14-week pregnant patient needs a contrast enhanced MRI of the brain for glioma. Would you give contrast, and if yes, which one?

5. An 8-week hypotensive pregnant patient with history of road traffic accident (RTA) and a distended belly has a positive focussed assessment with sonography for trauma (FAST) USG. What is the next best step in terms of imaging/ management?

6. A 24-week pregnant lady has suspected appendicitis and indeterminate USG. What is the next best step in terms of imaging/management?

STEPS TO BE TAKEN PRIOR TO EXAMINATION

- Always ask the last date of the menstrual cycle for all female patients in reproductive age.

- Confirm the pregnancy status and weeks of gestation. If unsure, a pregnancy test must be performed prior to the examination.
- If the patient is pregnant, the indication and the specific examination for the indication must be justified. Discuss each case with the referring physician and assess the risk–benefit ratio. Check whether USG or non-contrast MRI will provide the required information. Be factual while explaining to the patient regarding the need for the study, the available options if any, and the risk–benefit ratio.
- Providing lead shielding to wrap the pelvis of the pregnant patient during a non-pelvic CT may help the emotional well-being of the patient, but the dose to the uterus (primarily from internal scatter radiation) is not materially altered by this shielding.

RISKS RELATED TO RADIATION EXPOSURE

- Fetal radiation risks can be stochastic or deterministic. The ACR and International Committee on Radiological Protection (ICRP) have published a table of *in utero* radiation-induced deterministic effects in the fetus depending on the gestational age and the degree of radiation exposure (Table 3.1).[2]

  a. Fetal radiation doses below 50 mGy is not known to cause fetal toxicity.

  b. Radiation exposure up to 100 mGy should not be considered a reason for terminating a pregnancy as per ACR and ICRP.

  c. Radiation doses above 100 mGy may result in a 1% combined increased risk of organ malformation and the development of childhood cancer.

- **Radiation exposure per procedure is usually much lower than 50 mGy for even major diagnostic studies like PET/CT; so performing CT should be safe in pregnancy when indicated.** Please refer to Table 1.1 in Chapter 1 for the estimated radiation doses to adults from common imaging examinations.

Table 3.1: The ACR summary of suspected *in utero* induced deterministic effects published by the ICRP

Gestational age	Conception age	Radiation dose		
		<50 mGy (<5 rad)	50–100 mGy (5–10 rad)	>100 mGy (>10 rad)
0–2 weeks (0–14 days)	Before conception	None	None	None
3rd and 4th weeks (15–28 days)	1st–2nd weeks (1–14 days)	None	Probably none	Possible spontaneous abortion
5th–10th weeks (29–70 days)	3rd–8th weeks (15–56 days)	None	Potential effects are scientifically uncertain and probably too subtle to be clinically detectable	Possible malformations increase in likelihood as dose increases
11th–17th weeks (71–119 days)	9th–15th weeks (57–105 days)	None	Potential effects are scientifically uncertain and probably too subtle to be clinically detectable	Increased risk of deficits in IQ or mental retardation that increase in frequency and severity with increasing dose
18th–27th weeks (120–189 days)	16th–25th weeks (106–175 days)	None	None	IQ deficits not detectable at diagnostic doses
>27 weeks (>189 days)	>25 weeks (>175 days)	None	None	None applicable to diagnostic medicine

- In the first four weeks of gestation, fetal radiation exposure follows an all-or-none phenomenon. At high doses (>100 mGy), if there is any radiation toxicity to the fetus, it will kill the fledgling fetus leading to 'spontaneous' abortion. Otherwise, the fetus will survive without any pathologic or physiologic consequence on subsequent development.
- According to the consensus statements from the relevant major international organizations (National Council on Radiation Protection [NCRP], ICRP, Biologic Effects of Ionizing Radiation VII [BEIRVII], Centers for Disease Control and Prevention, ACR, and American Congress of Obstetricians and Gynecologists [ACOG]), **the risk of malignancy, miscarriage, or major malformations is negligible in fetuses exposed to 50 mGy or less.**

MAMMOGRAPHY DURING PREGNANCY

- The radiation dose from bilateral two view digital and film-screen mammography studies is less than 3 mGy. The estimated dose to the uterus is less than 0.03 µGy.
- Lead apron shielding may decrease the dose to the uterus by up to 50%.
- If a patient happens to undergo mammography before she is aware of her pregnancy status, she should be assured that the risk to the early fetus is very minimal, if any.
- Routine annual screening mammography is not performed during pregnancy.
- The sensitivity of mammography in detecting pregnancy-associated breast cancer is less than that of ultrasound. Hence, USG is preferred in these patients.

USE OF IV CONTRAST FOR CT IN PREGNANCY

- IV iodinated contrast is a category B drug as per the US Food and Drug Administration (FDA). This means that while no fetal risk/teratogenicity has been documented in animal studies, no controlled studies have been performed in pregnant women. To put things in perspective, other category B drugs include paracetamol, benadryl, and methyldopa (drug of choice for pregnancy-induced hypertension!). Thus, it is quite safe to use IV contrast in pregnancy.

- Although iodinated contrast agents can cause neonatal hypothyroidism if directly instilled into the amniotic sac, there are no reports of clinical sequelae induced by iodinated contrast agents administered IV.

- **However, the patient must be informed of the need to undergo neonatal thyroid screening in the first week post-delivery. This is anyway a part of the routine neonatal screening protocol.** Multiple studies have found no increased incidence of thyroid dysfunction in neonates exposed to IV contrast *in utero*, indicating that this risk is again more theoretical than real. Needless to say, the neonatal thyroid screening still needs to be routinely performed.

MRI DURING PREGNANCY

- The potential risk of heating effects from radiofrequency pulses and effects of acoustic noise on the fetus have not been proven. All major organizations deem 1.5T MRI to be safe for MRI in pregnancy.

- Prefer performing the MRI on a 1.5T magnet rather than a 3T magnet as safety on higher strength magnets has not been assessed rigorously as yet. However, no harm has been reported on 3T either.

- Studies have shown that the fetus can excrete, swallow, and reabsorb gadolinium into the GI tract with gadolinium remaining in the amniotic fluid indefinitely, because the half-life of gadolinium in the fetus is unknown. This leads to the potential risk of gadolinium dechelation and the fetus developing an NSF-like syndrome.

- The US FDA has classified gadolinium-based agents as category C drugs, meaning that animal studies have revealed adverse effects on the fetus (at supraclinical doses), but there have been no controlled studies in women.

- The ACR Guidance Document on Safe MRI Practices published in 2013 states that given the theoretical but potentially real risk of gadolinium toxicity to the fetus, a decision to give IV contrast should be based on an *overwhelming* clinical benefit for the patient outweighing this risk.

- A large retrospective study published in Journal of the American Medical Association (JAMA) in 2016 observed an increased risk of rheumatological, inflammatory or infiltrative skin conditions in children who were exposed to gadolinium in the first trimester, thus indicating that the ACR position is indeed valid.

- **If there is indeed an unavoidable need to perform a CE-MRI (say, in a patient with a brain tumor), preferably use Dotarem, Prohance, or Gadovist (stabler macrocyclic agents with lowest risk of NSF); else use Multihance (intermediate risk of NSF) in pregnant patients. Magnevist, Omniscan, and Optimark are contraindicated.**

- Do not administer gadolinium-based contrast agents in patients with renal impairment.

SELECTING THE APPROPRIATE STUDY FOR THE APPROPRIATE CLINICAL SCENARIO

- In general, prefer performing a USG or a non-contrast MRI if they would be able to answer the clinical question. However, remember that delayed diagnosis would usually cause more morbidity and mortality to the mother and fetus than performing an indicated CECT or even a CE-MRI, and decide appropriately on a case-by-case basis.

- Given that IV iodinated contrast is quite safe in pregnancy, if you decide to perform a CT study, it is better to perform it with IV contrast if indicated to avoid the need to repeat the study if the diagnostic information from the non-contrast scan is suboptimal.

- In patients with trauma, MRI has a very limited role. CECT is the investigation of choice given its speed, ability to cover the entire relevant body, and ability to detect fractures.

- Appendicitis in pregnant patients is often atypical in presentation and difficult to detect on USG. Furthermore, a delay in diagnosis or a negative laparotomy both lead to worsened maternal and fetal outcomes. Thus, fast and accurate diagnosis is important (clinical observation is not a good option).

- In cases of suspected appendicitis with indeterminate USG, prefer a non-contrast MRI if available. MRI has >90% sensitivity and specificity, a positive predictive value of 0.86, and **a negative predictive value of 0.99** (if we see a normal appendix on MRI, the patient does not have appendicitis 99% of the time). If MRI facilities are not available, perform a CECT instead.

- For patients with suspected pulmonary embolism, first ensure that the D-dimer levels are elevated. Prefer to first perform a lower limb Doppler to look for deep venous thrombosis. If negative, then it is appropriate to perform a CT pulmonary angiogram (CT PA) to rule out pulmonary embolism in the appropriate clinical scenario. Fleishner Society recommends CT PA over a V/Q (ventilator/perfusion) scan given that CT can provide additional information which may explain the patient's symptoms.

LACTATING PATIENTS

- According to the ACR Manual on contrast media, it should be safe for the mother and infant to continue breastfeeding after receiving iodinated or gadolinium-based contrast agents, but if the mother desires, she may choose to wait for 24 hours before resuming breastfeeding. This is irrespective of the renal status of the mother.

- ESUR concurs with ACR with regards to iodinated contrast media. However, ESUR guidelines advise stopping breastfeeding for 24 hours if high-risk gadolinium contrast agents (namely Optimark, Omniscan, and Magnevist) are used for CE-MRI.
- In a planned study, if the mother desires to withhold breastfeeding for 24 hours, she should be advised to pump breast milk beforehand. There is no value to withholding breastfeeding beyond 24 hours after contrast injection.
- In women older than 40 years old, mammography screening should resume approximately 3 months after cessation of lactation to allow the breast parenchyma to fully involute and return to baseline density.
- Lactating patients should be asked to nurse or pump immediately before undergoing mammography to decrease parenchymal density related to retained milk products as much as possible.

WHAT TO COUNSEL THE PREGNANT PATIENT

- Unless procedures with radiation risk are repeated during the course of pregnancy, none have a radiation dose higher than the absolute safe threshold of 50 mGy.
- Prefer using layman terms rather than technical terms to help them understand. For example, you may explain that radiation exposure by CT is much less than the dose of annual background radiation a person living in certain parts of Kerala (up to 70 mGy!).
- Always remind them that there remains a 15–20% chance of a miscarriage/anomaly associated with all routine pregnancies.
- For consent for IV contrast, explain and take a written informed consent which includes the following points: Need for the study and for IV contrast, possible other options explained, clinical information obtained will

affect treatment of mother and/or child, benefits out-weigh the risk, explanation about routine chance of miscarriage/anomaly, explanation about preemptive breast milk pumping (if she wishes to avoid lactation).

AT A GLANCE

- There is no risk of malignancy, miscarriage, or major malformations in fetuses exposed to 50 mGy or less, as per major international organizations including ICRP, NCRP, ACR, and ACOG. Given that one-time diagnostic radiation is less than half that cut-off, all diagnostic imaging modalities are safe to be used in pregnant women, but should be performed only if there is a relevant clinical indication, given the social and emotional issues involved and the general public and medical community perceptions of harm from radiation, even if scientifically non-existent.
- IV iodinated contrast is safe to use in pregnant/lactating patients. The theoretical risk of thyroid toxicity is also not demonstrated in multiple studies; however, a neonatal thyroid screening should be performed in all such patients as is the routine standard of care for every child.
- Gadolinium-based contrast media should be avoided in pregnancy unless there is an overwhelming clinical benefit (for example, in patients with a suspected brain tumor).
- Intermediate-risk and low-risk gadolinium contrast agents are safe to use in lactating patients as per both ACR and ESUR guidelines. With regards to high-risk gado-linium contrast agents, ACR deems them safe while ESUR advises to avoid breastfeeding for 24 hours.

Answers to Clinical Scenarios

Q1. *A 10-week pregnant lady with a single live fetus on a recent USG had a single phase CT abdomen at 4 weeks. How high is the risk of the baby developing a malformation due to the CT? Should she abort or not?*

Ans: Since the baby is alive, there is no risk of developing a malformation (radiation exposure is an all-or-none phenomenon in fetuses <4 weeks of age).

Q2. *A 14-week pregnant patient needs a CECT abdomen and pelvis. What should you be extremely worried about: Fetal radiation exposure, fetal renal toxicity, or fetal thyroid toxicity?*

Ans: There is no need to extremely worried about any of these. However, a routine neonatal thyroid screen must be performed.

Q3. *A 14-week pregnant patient needs an MRI pelvis for suspected AVN of hip. Your hospital has both a 1.5T MRI and a 3T MRI. Are both equally safe or would you prefer using one over the other?*

Ans: Prefer to perform the MRI on a 1.5T machine, though there is no evidence that there is any harm on a 3T machine. If the facility has only a 3T machine, it is fair to go ahead with scanning on a 3T scanner.

Q4. *A 14-week pregnant patient needs a CE-MRI of the brain for glioma. Would you give contrast, and if yes, which one?*

Ans: In this situation, the information that a CE-MRI can provide does represent overwhelming clinical benefit. CE-MRI may be performed using a macrocyclic agent.

Q5. *An 8-week hypotensive pregnant patient with history of RTA and a distended belly has a positive FAST USG. What is the next best step in terms or imaging/management?*

Ans: Perform CECT.

Q6. *A 24-week pregnant lady has suspected appendicitis and indeterminate USG. What is the next best step in terms of imaging/management?*

Ans: Perform non-contrast MRI.

Suggested Further Reading

1. ACR–SPR Practice Parameter for Imaging Pregnant or Potentially Pregnant Adolescents and Women with Ionizing Radiation. Available at https://www.acr.org/~/media/ACR/Documents/PGTS/guidelines/Pregnant_Patients.pdf?la= en.Accessed on 7.6.17.

2. American College of Radiology. Radiation Dose to Adults from Common Imaging Examinations. https://www.acr.org/~/media/ACR/Documents/PDF/QualitySafety/Radiation-Safety/Dose-Reference-Card.pdf. Accessed on 28.6.17

3. Baheti AD, Nicola R, Bennett GL, Bordia R, Moshiri M, Katz DS, Bhargava P.Magnetic Resonance Imaging of Abdominal and Pelvic Pain in the Pregnant Patient. MagnReson Imaging Clin N Am 2016; 24:403–17.

4. Wang PI, Chong ST, Kielar AZ, et al. Imaging of pregnant and lactating patients: part 1, evidence-based review and recommendations. AJR Am J Roentgenol 2012;198:778–84.

5. Wang PI, Chong ST, Kielar AZ, et al. Imaging of pregnant and lactating patients: part 2, evidence-based review and recommendations. AJR Am J Roentgenol 2012;198:785–92.

6. Wieseler KM, Bhargava P, Kanal KM, Vaidya S, Stewart BK, Dighe MK. Imaging in pregnant patients: examination appropriateness. Radiographics 2010;30:1215–29.

BIBLIOGRAPHY

1. ACR–SPR Practice Parameter for Imaging Pregnant or Potentially Pregnant Adolescents and Women with Ionizing Radiation. Available at https://www.acr.org/~/media/ACR/Documents/PGTS/guidelines/Pregnant_Patients.pdf?la=en. Accessed on 7.6.17.

2. McCollough CH, Schueler BA, Atwell TD, et al. Radiation exposure and pregnancy: when should we be concerned? *Radiographics* 2007;27:909–17.

3. Radiation Dose to Adults from Common Imaging Examinations. Accessed from https://www.acr. org/~/media/ACR/Documents/PDF/QualitySafety/Radiation-Safety/Dose-Reference-Card. pdf. Accessed on 28.7.17.

4. Ray JG, Vermeulen MJ, Bharatha A, Montanera WJ, Park AL. Association Between MRI Exposure During Pregnancy and Fetal and Childhood Outcomes. JAMA 2016; 316:952–61.

5. Wang PI, Chong ST, Kielar AZ, et al. Imaging of pregnant and lactating patients: part 1, evidence-based review and recommendations. *AJR Am J Roentgenol* 2012;198:778–84.

6. Wieseler KM, Bhargava P, Kanal KM, Vaidya S, Stewart BK, Dighe MK. Imaging in pregnant patients: examination appropriateness. *Radiographics* 2010;30:1215–29.

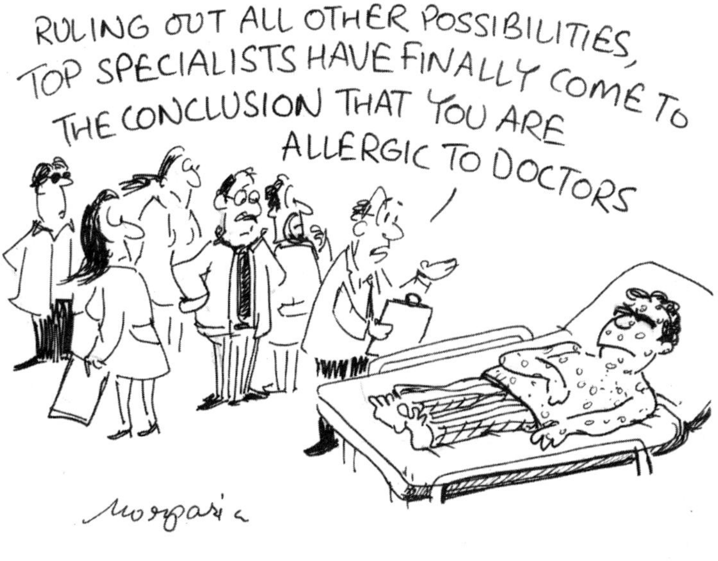
RULING OUT ALL OTHER POSSIBILITIES, TOP SPECIALISTS HAVE FINALLY COME TO THE CONCLUSION THAT YOU ARE ALLERGIC TO DOCTORS
Morparia

Chapter 4

Management of Contrast Reactions and Extravasation

Akshay Baheti, Sharad Maheshwari

Clinical Scenarios

1. A patient with history of mild contrast reaction (development of a few hives) comes for an appointment for an indicated contrast-enhanced CT. Should we do the study? If yes, should we give pre-medications?
2. A patient with history of moderate vasovagal reaction on the previous CT comes for an indicated repeat CECT. Should we do the study? If yes, should we give pre-medications?
3. A patient with history of a mild allergic contrast reaction comes for a repeat CECT, and tell you he has forgotten to take his premedication regimen. He asks whether he will certainly get a reaction again, and asks how likely it is that the reaction will be more severe? He wants to accordingly decide between delaying the scan for a day or taking the risk of doing the scan right away. What is your answer?
4. What is the role of thrombophobe in managing extravasation?

MANAGEMENT OF CONTRAST REACTIONS

Points to Note

- Contrast reactions can either be allergic-like or physiologic in etiology.
- If a patient develops a contrast reaction, apart from immediate treatment and patient care, the type of reaction should be identified and the reaction should be graded as mild, moderate or severe. The grading should be documented so as to help future management. Such a suggested grading system is given in Table 4.1.

Table 4.1: Classification of allergic-like contrast reactions

Mild	• Limited cutaneous reactions, e.g. few hives, mild pruritis, or transient flushing • Mild cutaneous edema • 'Itchy/scratchy' throat • Nasal congestion, sneezing, conjunctivitis
Moderate	• Diffuse urticaria (multiple hives) or pruritis • Moderate or severe erythema with stable vitals • Facial edema without dyspnea • Breathing problems such as wheezing, bronchospasm, throat tightness or hoarseness without dyspnea/none or mild hypoxia
Severe	• Diffuse erythema, with hypotension • Body/facial edema with dyspnea • Breathing problems such as wheezing, bronchospasm, throat tightness or hoarseness with dyspnea/ significant hypoxia • Anaphylactic shock

PREMEDICATION GUIDELINES FOR ALLERGIC-LIKE REACTIONS

- Premedication must be given for every patient with moderate or severe allergic-like reaction.
- For patients with history of mild allergic-like reaction, premedication is recommended by ACR but not necessary as per ESUR guidelines. Thus, different institutes may have different protocols. Either ways, if the patient has forgotten to take the premedication, she/he may be allowed to opt to undergo the CECT after appropriate counselling and informed consent, but after having been explained that the risk of recurrent reaction is approximately 8–25%, which is usually of the same severity as the prior one (in about 85% cases).
- Steroids should be given beginning at least 6 hours prior to the contrast (regardless of the route of steroid administration) whenever possible; a less recent steroid administration will not lead to a reduced risk of contrast reaction.

- Prefer to perform the scan with a radiologist around, and ensure that a code team (emergency medical team) is available.
- Avoid giving iodinated oral contrast in patients with history of moderate–severe allergy; instead use barium-based oral contrast.
- Although of no proven benefit, a different IV contrast from the one administered previously may be used.

PREMEDICATION REGIMENS

Elective (in order of preference)

1. Prednisone—50 mg by mouth at 13 hours, 7 hours, and 1 hour before study, plus diphenhydramine—50 mg intravenously, intramuscularly, or by mouth 1 hour before study (Greenberger regimen). When oral medication is not possible, replace prednisolone by 200 mg hydrocortisone.
2. Methylprednisolone—32 mg by mouth 12 hours and 2 hours before study, plus diphenhydramine—50 mg intravenously, intramuscularly, or by mouth 2 hours before study.

Emergency

Methylprednisolone 40 mg or hydrocortisone sodium succinate 200 mg intravenously 6 and 2 hours prior to the study plus diphenhydramine 50 mg IV 1 hour prior to contrast injection.

PHYSIOLOGIC REACTIONS

Physiologic reactions include nausea, vomiting, transient flushing, warmth, headache, dizziness, hypertension, isolated chest pain, vasovagal reaction (hypotension with bradycardia), arrhythmia, and convulsions.

Patients who have had prior physiologic reactions may be at a higher risk of a repeat reaction, but premedication is not indicated.

MANAGEMENT OF CONTRAST REACTIONS

- Detailing the management of acute contrast reactions is beyond the scope of this book. Basic guidelines are provided, *refer* to Flowchart 4.1 for details.

Flowchart 4.1: Management of acute reaction to contrast media

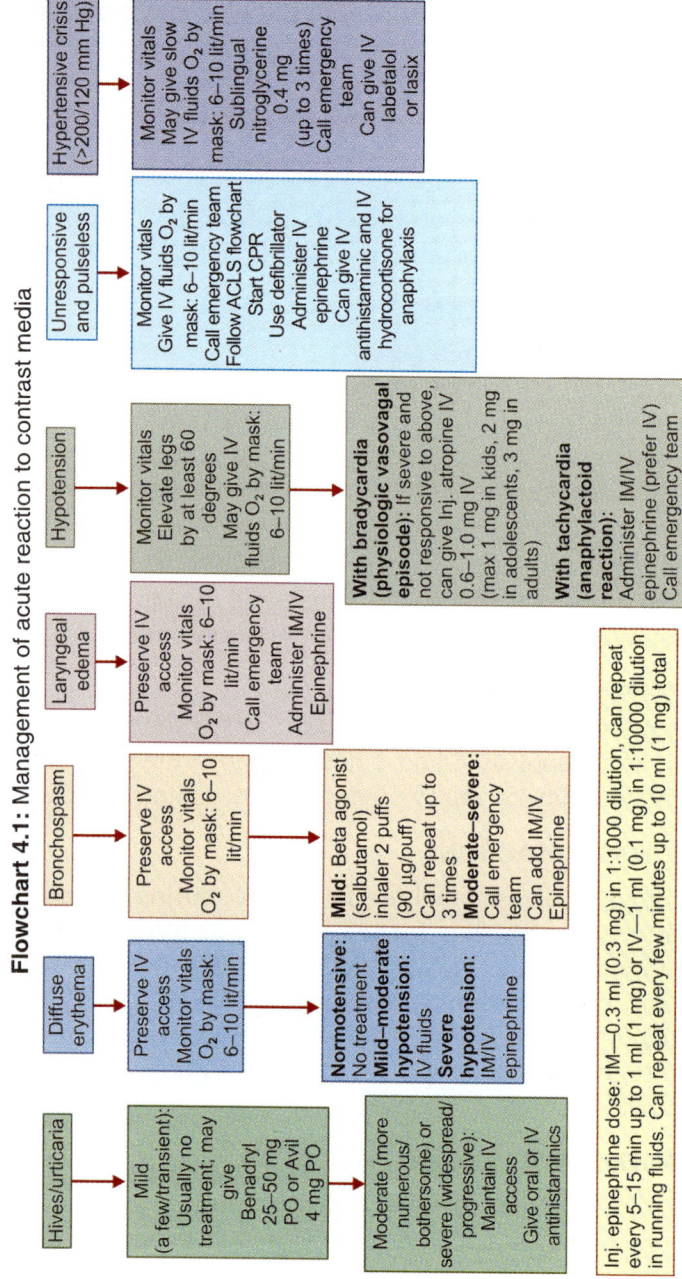

Hives/urticaria
- Mild (a few/transient): Usually no treatment; may give Benadryl 25–50 mg PO or Avil 4 mg PO
- Moderate (more numerous/ bothersome) or severe (widespread/ progressive): Maintain IV access Give oral or IV antihistaminics

Diffuse erythema
- Preserve IV access Monitor vitals O₂ by mask: 6–10 lit/min
- **Normotensive:** No treatment **Mild–moderate hypotension:** IV fluids **Severe hypotension:** IM/IV epinephrine

Bronchospasm
- Preserve IV access Monitor vitals O₂ by mask: 6–10 lit/min
- **Mild:** Beta agonist (salbutamol) inhaler 2 puffs (90 µg/puff) Can repeat up to 3 times **Moderate–severe:** Call emergency team Can add IM/IV Epinephrine

Laryngeal edema
- Preserve IV access Monitor vitals O₂ by mask: 6–10 lit/min Call emergency team Administer IM/IV Epinephrine

Hypotension
- Monitor vitals Elevate legs by at least 60 degrees May give IV fluids O₂ by mask: 6–10 lit/min
- **With bradycardia (physiologic vasovagal episode):** If severe and not responsive to above, can give Inj. atropine IV 0.6–1.0 mg IV (max 1 mg in kids, 2 mg in adolescents, 3 mg in adults) **With tachycardia (anaphylactoid reaction):** Administer IM/IV epinephrine (prefer IV) Call emergency team

Unresponsive and pulseless
- Monitor vitals Give IV fluids O₂ by mask: 6–10 lit/min Call emergency team Follow ACLS flowchart Start CPR Use defibrillator Administer IV epinephrine Can give IV antihistaminic and IV hydrocortisone for anaphylaxis

Hypertensive crisis (>200/120 mm Hg)
- Monitor vitals May give slow IV fluids O₂ by mask: 6–10 lit/min Sublingual nitroglycerine 0.4 mg (up to 3 times) Call emergency team Can give IV labetalol or lasix

Inj. epinephrine dose: IM—0.3 ml (0.3 mg) in 1:1000 dilution, can repeat every 5–15 min up to 1 ml (1 mg) or IV—1 ml (0.1 mg) in 1:10000 dilution in running fluids. Can repeat every few minutes up to 10 ml (1 mg) total

Observe patients with mild reaction for at least half an hour. Let them go home if the reaction is stable or improving, with instructions on identifying danger signs. They may take an antihistaminic at home if they get any delayed mild reactions

- One must be well prepared to manage any acute contrast reaction. An appropriate management algorithm must be present in every CT room along with a crash cart/ emergency cart.
- Radiologists should ideally have taken an advanced cardiac life support (ACLS) or at least a basic life support (BLS) course. An automated defibrillator must be handy, and the radiologist and support staff must be trained in its use.
- Immediately call the support staff in case of any moderate or severe contrast reaction and ask them to call the emergency team. **Elevate the patient's legs, begin oxygen, and take the patient's vitals immediately. Based on the pulse, one can differentiate between a vasovagal episode and an anaphylactoid reaction; begin management accordingly.**
- For mild reactions, simply monitoring the patient for 30 minutes along with counselling often suffices. An oral anti-histaminic may be prescribed if needed.

MANAGEMENT OF CONTRAST EXTRAVASATION

Points to Note

- IV contrast extravasation is an uncommon complication of contrast injection. Suggested classification and management of the same is provided in Table 4.2.
- The technician or nurse should be monitoring the first 10 sec of the contrast injection inside the console in every patient (an exception may be made for arterial phase injections).
- The frequency of extravasation is not related to the injection flow rate.
- Thrombophobe, glycerine magnesium sulphate, and injection hyaluronidase have no proven role in treating extravasation.
- Extravasation injury can worsen over time, as the inflammatory response to contrast can peak at 24–48 hours. Therefore, close clinical follow-up for several hours is essential in

moderate–severe cases. Patients can be sent home without follow-up only if the symptoms remain stable or improve. A documented follow-up phone call in 24–48 hours for all cases would be ideal.

- Clear instructions should be given to the patient to seek additional medical care, should there be any worsening of symptoms, skin ulceration, or the development of any neurologic or circulatory symptoms, including paresthesias.

Table 4.2: Classification and management of extravasation		
Severity	*Clinical signs*	*Management*
Mild	• No signs/symptoms • Only pain/swelling/mild erythema	None or limb elevation and cold compress
Moderate	• Moderate or severe erythema • Blistering • Moderate pain or swelling • All signs and symptoms must resolve within 2 weeks of the extravasation	Limb elevation, cold compress Call plastic services as indicated
Severe	• Unremitting pain and swelling • Limitations in extremity movement • Any extravasation which requires surgical intervention • Signs and symptoms last more than 2 weeks	Limb elevation, cold compress Call plastic services as indicated

WHEN TO CALL THE PLASTIC SURGEON

A plastic surgery reference is a good idea whenever there is any doubt in the mind of the radiologist about potential development of compartment syndrome. Plastic reference may be made in the following situations.

a. Extravasation volume is estimated to be almost the entire volume of contrast injection
b. Presence of skin blistering
c. There is possible altered tissue perfusion (as evidenced by delayed capillary refill time)
d. Pain at the extravasation site increases over time
e. There is a change in sensation at or adjacent to the extravasation site.
f. If there is any doubt because of any reason (even for mild extravasation), call the plastic surgeon.

AT A GLANCE

- Contrast reactions may be physiologic or allergic-like. Premedication is not required for patients with physiologic reactions, but is recommended in all cases of moderate–severe allergic-like reactions. Patients with mild allergic-like reactions may or may not be premedicated as per institutional preference.
- One must be well prepared to manage any acute contrast reaction. An appropriate management algorithm must be present in every CT room along with a crash cart/emergency cart.
- Any patient who has developed a contrast reaction must have the details documented on his/her file and must be explained about the utility of taking premedications in case of a future contrast-enhanced study.
- Mild contrast extravasation can be managed with hot/cold compresses and limb elevation. Patients must however be explained about the warning signs of compartment syndrome. Keep a low threshold for taking a plastic surgery consult.
- Thrombophobe, glycerine magnesium sulphate, and injection hyaluronidase have no proven role in managing extravasation.

Answers to Clinical Scenarios

Q1. *A patient with history of mild contrast reaction (development of a few hives) comes for an appointment for an indicated CECT. Should we do the study? If yes, should we give pre-medications?*

Ans: We should do the study. ACR recommends giving pre-medications in patients with history of mild allergic-like contrast reactions, while ESUR recommends giving premedication only in patients with moderate–severe reactions.

Q2. *A patient with history of moderate vasovagal reaction on the previous CT comes for an indicated repeat CECT. Should we do the study? If yes, should we give pre-medications?*

Ans: We should do the study. Premedication will not help as this is a physiological reaction.

Q3. A patient with history of a mild allergic contrast reaction comes for a repeat CECT, and tell you he has forgotten to take his premedication regimen. He asks whether he will certainly get a reaction again, and asks how likely it is that the reaction will be more severe? He wants to accordingly decide between delaying the scan for a day or taking the risk of doing the scan right away. What is your answer?

Ans: The risk of recurrent reaction is approximately 8–25%, which is usually of the same severity (in about 85% cases). So the patient will most likely not develop any reaction, or will develop a mild reaction. However, reiterate that he does have a higher than routine chance of developing a more severe reaction.

Q4. *What is the role of thrombophobe in managing extravasation?*

Ans: Thrombophobe has no proven role in managing extravasation.

Suggested Further Reading

1. Beckett KR, Moriarity AK, Langer JM. Safe Use of Contrast Media: What the Radiologist Needs to Know. Radiographics 2015; 35: 1738–50.
2. ESUR Contrast Media Guidelines version 8.1. Accessed from http://www.esur.org/guidelines.

3. Manual on Contrast Media v10.2. Accessed from https://www.acr.org/Quality-Safety/Resources/Contrast-Manual.

BIBLIOGRAPHY

1. Davenport MS, Cohan RH, Caoili EM, Ellis JH. Repeat contrast medium reactions in premedicated patients: frequency and severity. *Radiology* 2009;253:372–9.

2. Davenport MS, Cohan RH, Ellis JH. Contrast media controversies in 2015: imaging patients with renal impairment or risk of contrast reaction. *AJR Am J Roentgenol* 2015;204:1174–81.

3. ESUR Contrast Media Guidelines version 8.1. Accessed from http://www.esur.org/guidelines/ on 3.4.17.

4. Manual on Contrast Media v10.2. Accessed from https://www.acr.org/Quality-Safety/Resources/Contrast-Manual on 3.4.17.

5. Mervak BM, Davenport MS, Ellis JH, Cohan RH. Rates of Breakthrough Reactions in Inpatients at High Risk Receiving Premedication Before Contrast-Enhanced CT. *AJR Am J Roentgenol* 2015;205:77–84.

6. Wang CL, Cohan RH, Ellis JH, Adusumilli S, Dunnick NR. Frequency, management, and outcome of extravasation of nonionic iodinated contrast medium in 69,657 intravenous injections. *Radiology* 2007;243:80–7.

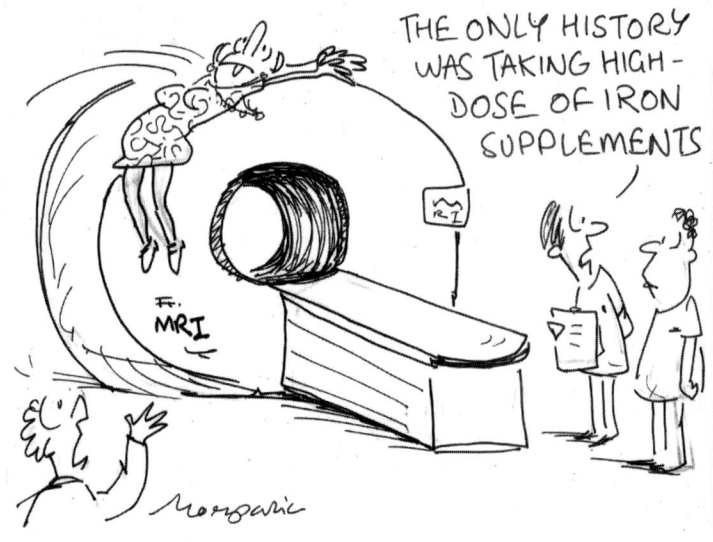

Chapter 5

Contraindications to MRI

Bhavin Jankharia, Akshay Baheti

INTRODUCTION

The list of absolute contraindications to MRI has steadily decreased over the past few years, with MRI compatible devices being regularly used across most procedures, and recent clinical work demonstrating the safety of MRI in patients with pacemakers and other cardiac devices.[1] Mrisafety.com is an excellent resource which provides relevant and reliable information on almost every available product with regards to MRI compatibility of metallic devices/implants, and should be used in case of any doubt. Always make it a point to check the make of the implanted device with the clinical notes/referring doctor in order to correctly confirm compatibility.

Basic Terminology with Respect MRI Compatibility

MRI safety terms were revised and standardized in 2005.[2]

MRI safe: No known hazard across all MRI environments.

MRI conditional: Demonstrated to pose no known hazards in specified MRI environments with specified conditions of use.

MRI unsafe: Known to be hazardous across all MRI environments.

Prior to 2005, the terms 'MRI safe' and 'MRI compatible' were used, often confusingly and interchangeably.[3] While both these terms were used for devices which had no known hazards related to MRI, an MRI safe device could potentially affect the quality of diagnostic information, while an MRI compatible device would not affect the quality of the diagnostic information nor have its operations affected by the MRI.[2] It is important to remember this as the new classification has not been retrospectively applied, and patients may come with devices labelled as per the old terminology.

Absolute Contraindications to MRI

Few absolute contraindications to MRI remain. These include:

1. Presence of a mobile internal metallic foreign body, such as a metallic foreign body in the ocular vitreous or a bullet in the abdomen (peritoneum).
2. Cochlear implant remains a relatively absolute contra-indication, although certain newer MRI conditional implants are now available.[4]
3. Subcutaneous insulin pumps: These need to be removed prior to the MRI.[5]
4. Cardiac pacemakers are not an absolute contraindication any longer, although the relevant technician must come over to alter the pacemaker settings for the MRI, and the scan must be performed with a ready emergency team.[6] Many new cardiac pacing systems are now MR condi-tional anyway, and a lot of recent evidence suggests that, particularly in non-pacemaker dependent patients, it is probably safe to perform the MRI in controlled settings.[1,6] Guidelines published by the ACR, American Heart Associa-tion and the European Society of Cardiology are available online to guide on performing an MRI in such patients.

For practical purposes, almost all other devices are safe. These include: Metallic bony implants, cardiac valves, aneurysm clips (even in an early postoperative patient), and stents. Of course, it is the duty of the radiologist to confirm the make of the device and clarify its status with respect to

MRI safety directly with the device literature or using mrisafety.org.

Patients with tattoos, permanent cosmetics or make-up which may contain ferromagnetic substances can safely undergo MRI (although they may cause artifacts), with any side-effects being rare and usually transient. The patients must be informed that they may get a warm or tingling sensation, and that they must call the technician/radiologist immediately should that happen. A close watch should be kept on such patients, and a cold compress may be kept handy as a precaution.[7]

REFERENCES

1. Russo RJ, Costa HS, Silva PD, et al. Assessing the Risks Associated with MRI in Patients with a Pacemaker or Defibrillator. N Engl J Med 2017;376:755–64.

2. Terminology with Regard to Magnetic Resonance Imaging (MRI) and Implants and Devices. http://www.mrisafety.com/Safety Infov.asp?SafetyInfoID=259. Accessed on 3.8.17.

3. Shellock FG, Crues JV, 3rd. MR Safety and the American College of Radiology White Paper. AJR Am J Roentgenol 2002;178:1349–52.

4. Cochlear Implants. http://www.mrisafety. com/Safety-Infov.asp?SafetyInfoID=170. Accessed on 5.8.2017.

5. Insulin pumps. http://www.mrisafety.com/SafetyInfov.asp?SafetyInfoID=271. Accessed on 5.8.2017.

6. Cardiac Pacemakers, Implantable Cardioverter Defibrillators (ICDs), and Cardiac Monitors. http://www.mrisafety.com/SafetyInfov.asp?SafetyInfoID=167. Accessed on 5.8.2017.

7. Tattoos, Permanent Cosmetics, and Eye Makeup. http://www.mrisafety.com/SafetyInfov.asp?SafetyInfoID=228. Accessed on 5.8.2017.

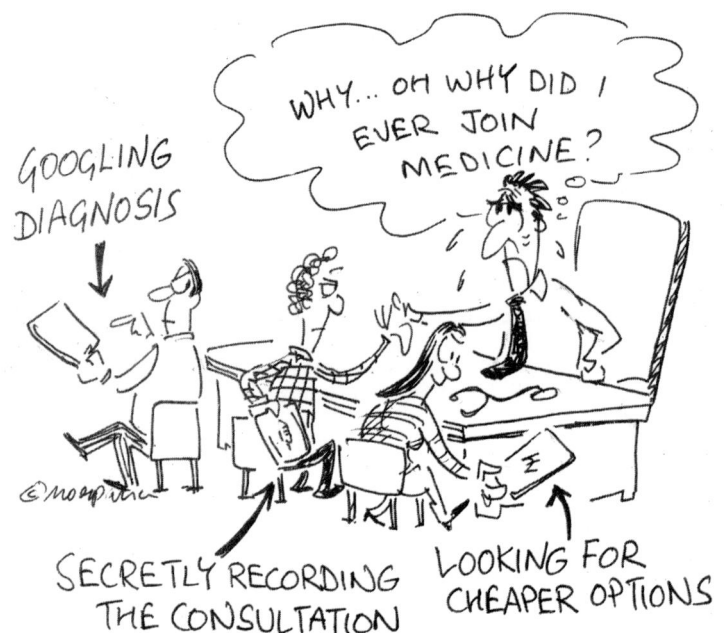

Chapter 6

Obtaining Consent: Current Status

Bhavin Jankharia, Akshay Baheti

A. INFORMED CONSENT FOR IV CONTRAST: CURRENT STATUS

INTRODUCTION

In the medical field, consent is often implied when the risk of adverse effects is low, and express when the risks are high. Both verbal and written consent are accepted forms of express consent. In diagnostic radiology in India, written informed consent is usually obtained before a contrast-enhanced study in most practices due to the risk of developing a contrast-related complication. This chapter discusses the various international guidelines on this issue. The authors have written an article on this topic in Indian Journal of Radiology and Imaging (IJRI), and the chapter is based on the same.[1]

Contrast-associated Risks

The common contrast-associated risks include contrast reaction or extravasation (<1% incidence each), and contrast-induced nephropathy or post-contrast acute kidney injury (AKI).[2] However, majority of the contrast reactions are mild, with deaths being very rare. A Japanese study of almost 170,000 patients receiving nonionic contrast reported a single death, which was also not definitely attributable to the contrast injection.[3] Similarly, post-contrast AKI is also uncommon, with recent literature proving that contrast is at worst a mild risk factor for nephropathy (*refer* to Chapter 2 for more details on this).[2, 4] In current practice, patients with poor renal function anyway do not receive IV contrast in most cases, thus making this point moot.

Based on this data, the ACR, Society of Pediatric Radiology (SPR) and Society of Interventional Radiology (SIR) state that IV contrast has a relatively low incidence of adverse events and may be exempted from the need for informed consent.[2,5] The guidelines however do mention that the consent policy of the institute should be based on state law, institutional and departmental policies, and local community practices. The Royal College of Radiology also states that implied consent suffices in very low-risk procedures.[6]

Alternative to Written Informed Consent

1. Unlike its counterparts, the IRIA unfortunately has not issued guidelines on this issue.

2. A patient information sheet explaining potential risks to the patient in a language they understand is a promising alternative, used widely across the world for the purposes of contrast injection.

3. A typical patient information sheet will explain the procedure, its potential risks, and ask questions to determine the patient's risk of developing a contrast related complication (history of prior contrast allergy, diabetes, renal disease, etc). Importantly, the patient is informed that if there are any queries, a radiologist is available to answer them. A signature may be obtained from the patient at the end of the sheet depending upon institutional policy.

4. A well-written patient information sheet in simple language can inform the patient in much more detail about the study, answer most of his/her questions, and alleviate procedure related anxiety.[7, 8] It is important to use lay language (for example, use 'dye' instead of 'contrast') so that the patient understands the information well. A positive risk factor (e.g. history of contrast allergy

or raised creatinine) should always lead to a radiologist-patient conversation. A sample format for a patient information sheet with signature is provided below.

Medicolegal Safety

1. Given our busy practices, it is difficult, if not impossible, for a radiologist to personally obtain consent in every case. The job often gets relegated to a technician, nurse, or even the receptionist. Many of them usually do not have any formal training on this issue for medicolegal purposes. A well-written patient information sheet with signature will provide more information to the patient in an easy to understand language.

2. To look for parallels in other medical specialties, a drug like penicillin (which has a much higher rate of anaphylaxis) is usually administered without obtaining written informed consent in most practices.

3. To the best of the authors knowledge, there is no legal precedent specific to radiology on this issue, neither in India nor in countries where written informed consent is not obtained. The only exception is a recent judgement given by the Delhi Consumer Forum in a case of death due to possible contrast reaction.[9] However, the judgement was given against the hospital because there was no doctor present to supervise the procedure and handle the reaction, and the hospital was ruled to have attempted to manipulate medical records to tamper with the time of death. This again underscores the fact that what is more important than a patient signature is adequate preparedness to handle a contrast reaction appropriately.

The Road Ahead

1. We believe that the patient information sheet with signature is a great potential tool to allow the patient to make an informed decision in its true spirit.

2. A radiologist however does need to be available for answering any questions the patient may have, besides of

course managing potential reactions. Importantly, written informed consent should be obtained in all high-risk patients.

3. The IRIA should take the initiative and give specific guidelines as also possibly a model patient information sheet with signature.

REFERENCES

1. Baheti AD, Thakur MH, Jankharia B. Informed Consent in Diagnostic Radiology Practice: Where do we Stand? Indian J Radiol Imaging (*in press*).
2. ESUR Contrast Media Guidelines version 8.1. Accessed from http://www.esur.org/guidelines/on 3.4.17.
3. Katayama H, Yamaguchi K, Kozuka T, Takashima T, Seez P, Matsuura K. Adverse reactions to ionic and nonionic contrast media. A report from the Japanese Committee on the Safety of Contrast Media. Radiology 1990;175: 621–8.
4. Davenport MS, Cohan RH, Ellis JH. Contrast media controversies in 2015: imaging patients with renal impairment or risk of contrast reaction. AJR Am J Roentgenol 2015;204:1174–81.
5. Kanda T, Ishii K, Kawaguchi H, Kitajima K, Takenaka D. High signal intensity in the dentate nucleus and globus pallidus on unenhanced T1-weighted MR images: relationship with increasing cumulative dose of a gadolinium-based contrast material. Radiology 2014;270:834–41.
6. Manual on Contrast Media v10.2. Accessed from https://www.acr.org/Quality-Safety/Resources/Contrast-Manual on 3.4.17.
7. Coyne CA, Xu R, Raich P, et al. Randomized, controlled trial of an easy-to-read informed consent statement for clinical trial participation: a study of the Eastern Cooperative Oncology Group. J Clin Oncol 2003;21:836–42.
8. Davis TC, Holcombe RF, Berkel HJ, Pramanik S, Divers SG. Informed consent for clinical trials: a comparative study of standard versus simplified forms. J Natl Cancer Inst 1998;90:668–74.
9. Allergic Reaction to CT Contrast: Batra Hospital to pay ` 8 lakh for negligence, tampering records. Accessed from http://medical-dialogues.in/allergic-reaction-to-ct-contrast-batra-hospital-to-rs-8-lakh-for-negligence-tampering-records/on 30.9.2017.

Know Your CT Contrast

What is a contrast injection and why do I need it?

Your doctor has asked for a CT scan using intravenous contrast (dye). This dye helps us provide more useful information for your treatment.

What are the risks involved?

Overall, contrast injections are very safe. However, there are always some small risks with every injection or medication. We are well trained and well prepared to treat these risks.

- Allergic reaction to contrast: The risk of this happening is <1%. The reaction is usually mild; however, 1 in 2500 patients may develop a more severe reaction. Our staffs are well trained to treat these. Very rarely, a death has occurred (1 out of 1.7 lakh patients) due to contrast allergy.

- Leakage of contrast during injection (<1% risk). The leakage is usually mild and self-limited.

  It may however rarely cause severe pain and need emergency surgery.

- Patients with pre-existing kidney disease may be at risk for kidney injury.

- Patients with myasthenia gravis might be at a slightly higher risk for experiencing disease worsening.

- Traditionally, patients with certain rare diseases like multiple myeloma, sickle cell disease, or pheochromocytoma were considered to be at a higher risk for IV contrast; however this is not proven.

	YES	NO
Please answer the following questions to assess your risk of developing a complication (check the appropriate column)		
Are you pregnant, or is there any chance that you might be pregnant?		
Have you had contrast allergy in the past?		
Do you have active asthma right now?		
Do you have kidney disease (kidney cancer, previous kidney surgery, have a single kidney)?		
Are you on dialysis?		
Do you take diabetes medicines*?		

*We need to know if you are taking any diabetes medicine which contains metformin.

If you have any queries or additional questions regarding your exam, one of us is available to answer them. Please feel free to discuss any questions with us prior to your study.

Your signature on this form indicates that you have read and understood the information provided in this form, authorize and consent to the performance of this procedure, and have had a chance to ask relevant questions.

Patient   Relative/Guardian   Relation with patient
Name & Signature   Name & Signature
                        (if patient is a minor)

_____   _____

_____

Name and Signature of Technologist/Nurse/Radiologist while accepting the form:

Sign: _____   Date : _____

B. INFORMED CONSENT FOR IMAGE-GUIDED INTERVENTION: HOW DO WE DO IT

INTRODUCTION

Image-guided interventional procedures require obtaining express informed consent as per various international guidelines.[1,2] Unfortunately, while our radiology training programs are excellent in creating proficient clinical radiologists, issues like interacting appropriately with patients and obtaining consent methodically are not focused upon in most residency programs, and usually the residents do not have the time to develop these important skills, due to the busy patient load.

In this chapter, we try to provide a basic 10-step framework on obtaining informed consent for any image-guided procedure. In its essence, obtaining consent means ensuring

a. that the patient and the treating radiologist develop a rapport and a level of trust,

b. that the patient understands the basic details about the procedure

c. that the patient understands the potential risks and complications (and perhaps their management), and

d. that basically the patient believes that he/she is in good hands.

Thus, while the details and fine print about the consent document are important, the manner of approaching and talking to the patient are equally, if not more important.

We wish to clarify that this is just a basic outline of 'must talk about' points during the process of obtaining informed consent. The process can (and indeed must) be individualized depending on the procedure and the patient. One way of taking consent has been highlighted in a video available at https://www.youtube.com/watch?v=fqWBv 0s7mio.

Steps and Points to follow while Obtaining Consent

1. Speak in a language that the patient is comfortable with. Confirm this at the beginning before starting the process of obtaining consent.

2. Remember that the procedure is being performed on the patient and not his/her relatives. Thus, focus on the patient while obtaining consent (even though the decision maker might appear to be the son/daughter/husband, etc.). If the patient develops trust in you and cooperates well during the procedure later on, your job will become much easier.

3. Begin the consent by acknowledging the patient and his/her relatives. As a policy, we do not allow more than 2–3 relatives along with the patient during obtaining consent. Clarify the relations between everyone. Maintain eye contact and smile while doing this. This helps develop rapport and a level of trust.

4. Introduce yourself and your team (the nurse/anesthetist, etc.). Explain your skill set, experience, and professional qualification in brief. This subconsciously reassures the patient that there is a well-oiled unit ready to care of him/her.

5. Give the patient an approximate timeline of how things will go. Give him/her an idea of when is the procedure expected to begin, how long will the procedure approximately take, and what are the immediate next steps that will happen (IV line, anesthesia, taking the patient in the CT room/intervention suite, etc.). If things are uncertain, state that and assure them that someone from the team will get back to them within a stipulated time period to give an update.

6. Explain the details of the procedure step-by-step in simple language. If the procedure is complex, you may also draw a simple diagram for help. Include practical points like the tingling which many experience during local anesthesia infiltration or the loud click of the

biopsy gun, which could otherwise make the patient uneasy. Explain relevant finer points as for example the need to obtain multiple biopsy samples.

7. Explain the potential common and serious complications to the patient. For example, in case of a lung biopsy, explain the possibility of bleeding, infection, and pneumothorax, as also the possibility of a negative biopsy. Give percentages to reassure that these complications are uncommon, wherever relevant. Clarify that your team is well equipped to handle any complications.

8. Explain your expectations from the patient. For example, patients need to understand the need to not make abrupt movements or to touch any part of the sterile field. Similarly, for lung biopsies, the patient needs to realize that he/she needs to take a similar volume of breath every time.

9. Confirm that the patient has understood everything and encourage them to ask any doubts or queries. Clarify that you are always available for answering questions which might pop up subsequently.

10. End by thanking the patient and the relatives for their support and cooperation, and explaining that someone from the team will meet after the procedure to explain the post-procedure steps.

REFERENCES

1. ACR–SIR–SPR practice parameter on informed consent for image-guided procedures, Revised 2016 (Resolution 17).

2. Standards for patient consent particular to radiology, Second edition, 2015. The Royal College of Radiologists.

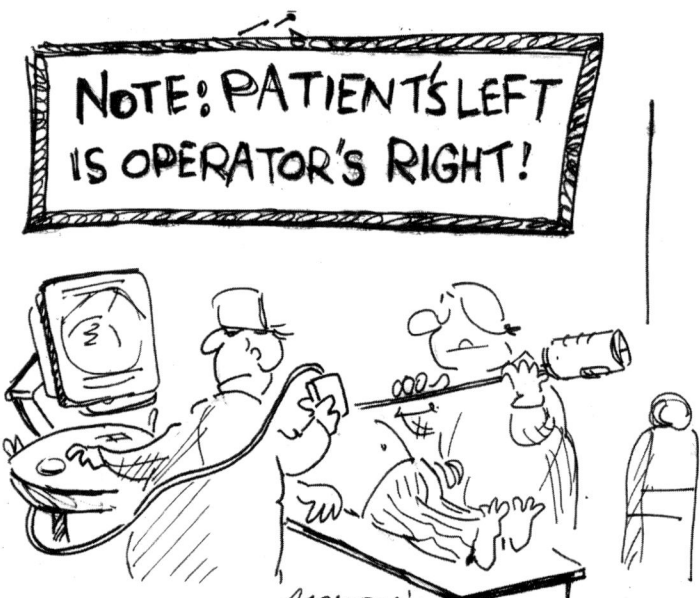

Chapter 7

Biopsy Checklist: What to Confirm before Inserting the Needle

Akshay Baheti, Bhavin Jankharia,

INTRODUCTION

The checklist is a commonly used tool for improving quality and safety standards in many industries, the airline industry being the most famous example.[1] Checklists have been proven to lead to improved adherence to the prescribed process and reduce errors and oversights. To imbibe the culture of using checklists for surgeries, the World Health Organization (WHO) published a surgical safety checklist for use at three time points during the peri-operative period: Before anesthesia, before the skin incision, and before the patient leaves the operating room.[2] Use of this checklist in eight hospitals across the world led to significant improvement in the rate of postoperative complications (from 11 to 7%), with the non-cardiac surgery patient mortality almost halving from 1.5 to 0.8%,[3] thus conclusively proving the valuable role a checklist can play in the medical field. One important practice in implementing the checklist is that any member of the team (i.e. including paramedics such as the nurse) can check it, thus empowering everyone in the team to catch and point out discrepancies.[1]

Although less invasive than surgery, both diagnostic and therapeutic interventional procedures do pose significant risks to the patient. A few checklists such as the Radiologic Patient Safety System (RADPASS) already exist.[4] This 27-item checklist has been found to reduce deviations from the optimum process from 24 to 5%, and reduce postponement or cancellation of intervention from 10 to 0%; an extraordinary success indeed.[5] We provide a suggested 11-item checklist for use before performing any diagnostic radiology intervention. This has been developed based on personal experience, feedback from other medical professionals, as also checklists used elsewhere. The checklist should be used at three time-points; before the patient is taken in the biopsy/intervention room, before beginning the procedure (before cleaning and draping the patient), and after the procedure is over. The checklist is by no means exhaustive, and may be modified as per institutional practices and the procedure itself. However, we hope this will serve as a basic template to work on to create personalized checklists in various institutes.

Procedure planning/preparation (to be completed by a radiologist before taking the patient in the room)

	Yes	No
1. Review original order for the biopsy/ intervention and its indication		
2. Allergies reviewed (specially related to contrast and anesthesia, if they are going to be used)		
3. Blood thinners/anticoagulants stopped appropriately and PT-INR/aPTT are normal[6] (Table 7.1)		
4. Clarified which samples to be taken and for what investigations*		
5. Any extra/special equipment or precautions needed for the procedure (e.g. for a patient who has HIV or HCV)		

Signature: **Date:**   **Time:**

* Whether the sample needs to be taken in formalin or saline or both; biopsy has to be sent for fungal or bacterial cultures or TB testing, etc., more samples needed for potential molecular testing as in EGFR/ALK testing for lung cancer

Before starting the procedure (time out) (to be completed by any person of the team)

	Yes	No
1. Correct patient, site/side, and procedure		
2. Written informed consent has been obtained		
3. Appropriate bottles ready for storing specimen		

Signature: **Date:**   **Time:**

Post-procedure (to be completed by any person of the team)

	Yes	No
1. Specimens labelled correctly and sent off		
2. Post-procedure orders written by the radiologist		
3. Post-procedure report given to the sister/doctor in the waiting room/ward		

Signature: **Date:**   **Time:**

Table 7.1: CIRSE guidelines for evaluation and management of bleeding risk in patients undergoing percutaneous biopsy[6]			
	Low (category 1)	*Moderate (category 2)*	*High (category 3)*
Risk of bleeding			
Type of biopsy	Superficial (thyroid, lymph nodes)	Lung, chest wall, intra-abdominal	Renal
Laboratory test			
INR	Recommended for patients receiving warfarin or liver diseases	Recommended	Routinely recommended
aPTT	Recommended for	Recommended for	Recommended for

Contd.

Table 7.1: CIRSE guidelines for evaluation and management of bleeding risk in patients undergoing percutaneous biopsy[6] (Contd.)

	Low (category 1)	*Moderate (category 2)*	*High (category 3)*
	patients receiving IV unfractioned heparin	patients receiving IV unfrac-tioned heparin	patients receiving IV unfractioned heparin
Platelet count	Not routinely recommended	Not routinely recommended	Routinely recommended
Hematocrit	Not routinely recommended	Not routinely recommended	Routinely recommended
Management			
INR	>2.0: Threshold for treatment	Correct to <1.5	Correct to <1.5
aPTT	No consensus	No consensus	Stop or reverse heparin for values >1.5 × control
Platelet count	Transfusion for counts <50,000/μl	Transfusion for counts <50,000/μl	Transfusion for counts <50,000/μl
Hematocrit	No recomm-ended thre-shold for transfusion	No recomm-ended thre-shold for transfusion	No recomm-ended threshold for transfusion
Drugs			
Clopidogrel	Withhold for 5 days before the procedure	Withhold for 5 days before the procedure	Withhold for 5 days before the procedure
Aspirin	Do not withhold	Do not withhold	Withhold for 5 days before the procedure

Contd.

Table 7.1: CIRSE guidelines for evaluation and management of bleeding risk in patients undergoing percutaneous biopsy[6] (Contd.)

LMWH	Withhold one dose before the procedure	Withhold one dose before the procedure	Withhold for 24 hours or up to two doses before the procedure
New oral anti-coagulants	Do not withhold	Withhold for 2–3 days before the procedure	Withhold for 3 days before the procedure

CIRSE: Cardiovascular and Interventional Radiological Society of Europe; INR: International normalized ratio; aPTT: Activated partial thromboplastin time; LMWH: Low molecular weight heparin.

REFERENCES

1. Gawande A. The Checklist Manifesto: How to get Things Right. New York: Metropolitan Books; 2010.
2. World Health Organization guidelines for safe surgery: safe surgery saves lives http://wwww hoint/patientsafety/safesurgery/tools_resources/9789241598552/en/Accessed on 17617.
3. Haynes AB, Weiser TG, Berry WR, et al. A surgical safety checklist to reduce morbidity and mortality in a global population. N Engl J Med 2009;360:491–9.
4. Rafiei P, Walser EM, Silberzweig JE, Nikolic B. Checklists for Image-guided Interventions. AJR Am J Roentgenol 2016:1–5.
5. Koetser IC, de Vries EN, van Delden OM, Smorenburg SM, Boermeester MA, van Lienden KP. A checklist to improve patient safety in interventional radiology. Cardiovasc Intervent Radiol 2013;36:312–9.
6. Veltri A, Bargellini I, Giorgi L, Almeida PAMS, Akhan O. CIRSE Guidelines on Percutaneous Needle Biopsy (PNB). Cardiovascular and Interventional Radiology. 2017 Oct; 40(10):1501–13.

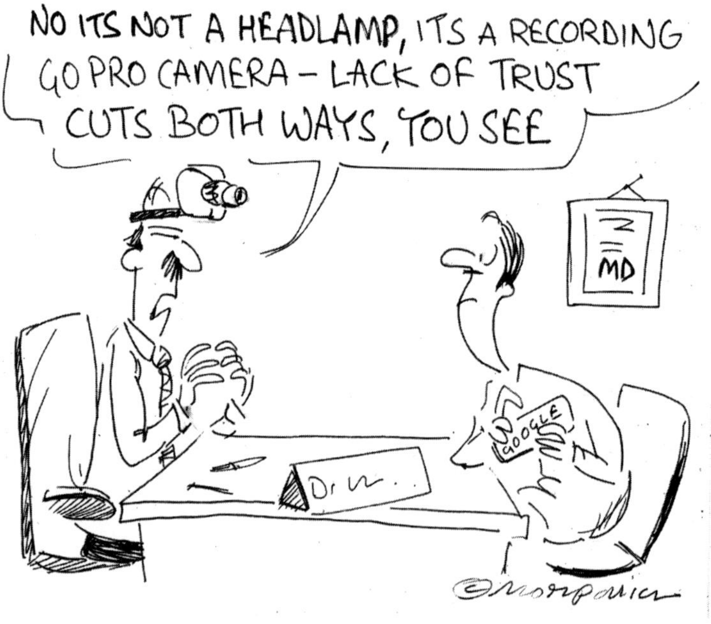
NO ITS NOT A HEADLAMP, ITS A RECORDING GO PRO CAMERA – LACK OF TRUST CUTS BOTH WAYS, YOU SEE
MD
GOOGLE

Chapter 8

Patient Rights and 'Un-Rights'

Bhavin Jankharia

It is a good idea in today's day and age to understand that patients have certain rights that come with getting a radiology study done. Some of these are legal, some ethical and moral, and some based on the standard of care at this point in time.

In such scenarios, it helps to understand these and to sensitize the staff and all those involved in making sure that these are not violated. Given the rate of angst being shown by patients against medical personnel, it helps to maintain a certain standard of care to prevent unwanted accidents and incidents from occurring.

At the same time, patients and relatives also need to follow a set of rules and behave appropriately; these are also listed.

Rights

1. *To meet a doctor prior to the study*

    If a patient has a question related to the study being done, he/she has every right to be able to speak to a doctor to get all his/her queries sorted out.

2. *Get an explanation about the procedure and possible risks, including those related to contrast*

    While a patient information sheet should suffice in most instances, if the patient wants more information from the doctor in attendance, that should be taken care of (*see* Chapter 6A)

3. *Get a full informed consent prior to an interventional procedure*

There is no questioning the fact that no patient should be taken up for any interventional procedure without a full informed consent (*see* Chapter 6B).

4. *To have access to a printed price list*

One major reason for the dwindling faith in doctors and the medical system is the lack of transparency in the pricing of a test. A printed price list displayed on the reception desk goes a long way in allaying patient apprehension about being overcharged. While there is no legal requirement at present, our experience has been that this can only be useful.

5. *To meet a doctor to discuss the report*

Again, this goes without saying. Any patient has the right to discuss his/her report findings. However, as discussed in the next section, we can make it very clear to the patient that we are not qualified to discuss management options, which should be done by their referring doctor.

6. *To have soft copy images on CD, USB and/or to have soft copy web access*

In today's day and age of volume studies with large data sets, it would be a travesty if all that the patient has is a set of films, many of them with matchbox-sized images, printed 30–40 per film. Every patient has an ethical right to all his/her volume data sets, preferably on CD or USB. Online access is also fine. This also allows other radiologists and physicians/surgeons to review the images for multiple opinions as well as to plan procedures, surgeries, do their own 3D and other similar reconstructions, amongst other uses.

Un-Rights

1. *Cannot shout, or abuse the staff*

We have a very low threshold of tolerance for staff abuse. The moment a patient raises his/her voice, they are told to cool it or to leave the premises. We have a series of cartoons displayed throughout our premises, currently only in English. We also have closed circuit television cameras (CCTVs) in all public areas to ensure that all such incidents are recorded for future verification.

2. *Bargain about the price*
   This has to be discouraged, because it leads to a sense that the prices are not fixed, that these are open to discussion and also enables other patients waiting around to start bargaining. This is just a bad way to manage any business/practice.

3. *Raise questions about the indication for the study and/or ask questions related to management after the report*
   As a rule, radiologists are not qualified to discuss management options, though there will always be exceptions, depending on expertise, place of work, indication for imaging, etc.

ANTI-ABUSE CARTOONS

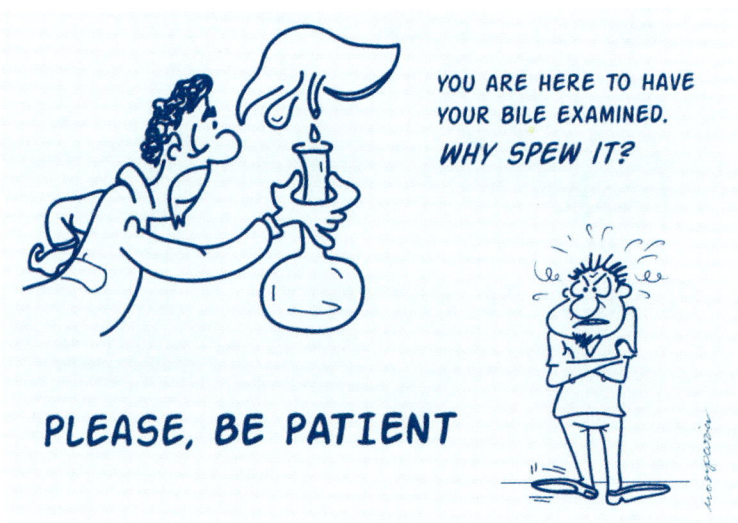

YOU ARE HERE TO HAVE YOUR BILE EXAMINED. *WHY SPEW IT?*

PLEASE, BE PATIENT

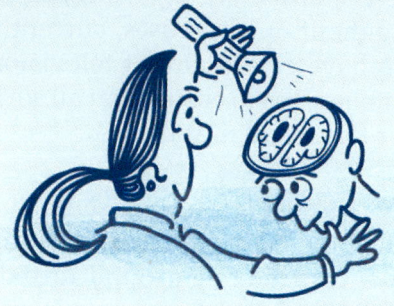

YOU ARE HERE TO GET
YOUR HEAD SCANNED.
WHY LOSE IT?

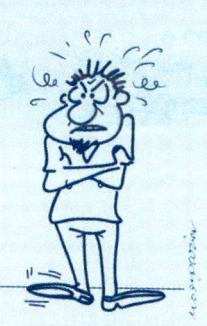

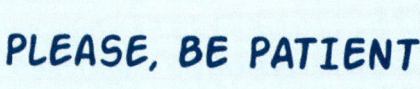

PLEASE, BE PATIENT

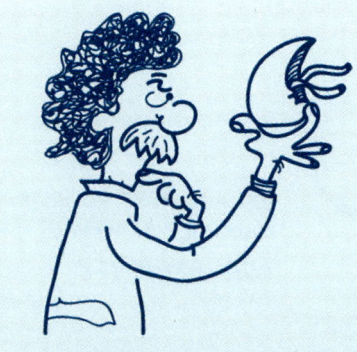

YOU ARE HERE TO GET
YOUR SPLEEN CHECKED.
WHY VENT IT?

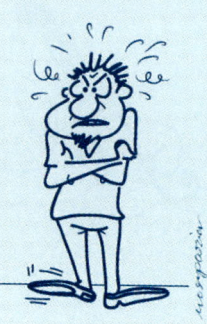

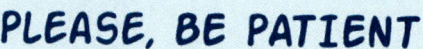

PLEASE, BE PATIENT

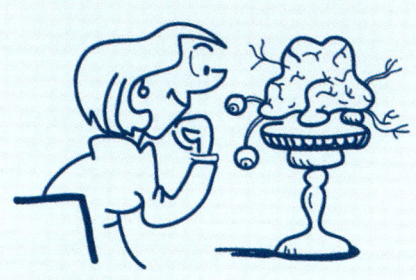

YOU ARE HERE TO GET
YOUR NERVES TESTED.
WHY GET ON OURS?

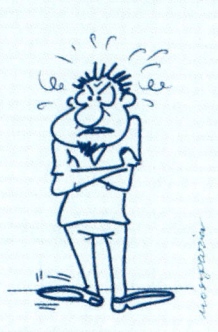

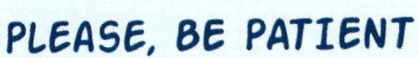

PLEASE, BE PATIENT

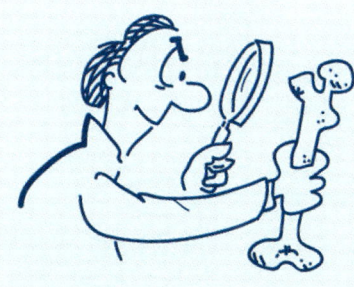

YOU ARE HERE TO GET
YOUR SKELETON STUDIED.
WHY PICK A BONE WITH US?

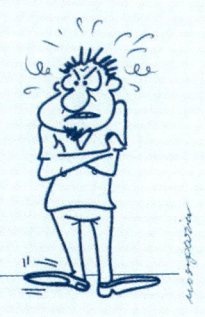

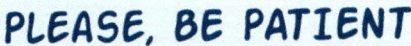

PLEASE, BE PATIENT

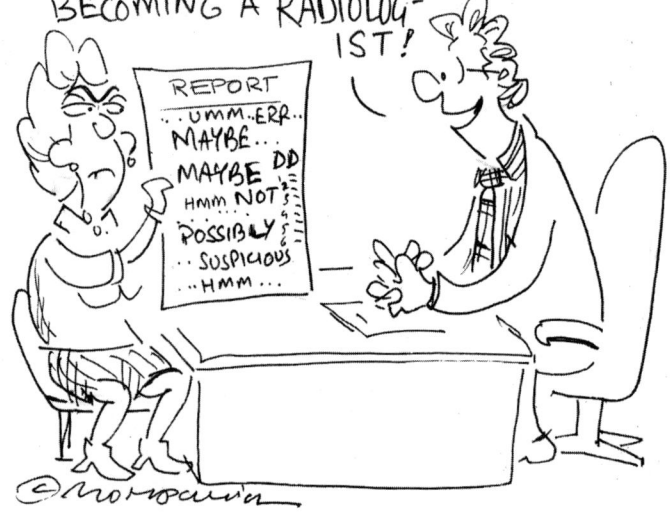

Chapter 9

Reports—Do's and Don'ts

Bhavin Jankharia

1. A 50-year-old man with a prior history of carcinoma rectum comes for CT abdomen. There is recurrence. The report is issued. He comes back 2 days later, requesting us to delete the statement mentioning comparison with the last CT scan. What do you do?

   The referring doctor calls and requests you to help. What do you do?

2. A 20-year-old lady comes for CT chest. By mistake, the report mentions 20-year-old male. They want the mistake rectified. What do you do?

3. A 60-year-old man with a right-sided cerebral mass has an MRI done. The report mentions left-sided. He comes back for rectification. What do you do?

4. A patient wants the study backdated so that she can avail insurance benefits. What do you do?

5. A patient comes for screening for migration to the Gulf. The CT scan shows a focal area of fibrosis in the right lower lobe. This is mentioned in the report. A well-wisher doctor calls and asks to remove this and to call it normal. What do you do?

6. A patient, let's say "Neha Gharda", gets an USG done. She comes back 3 days later saying, please change my name to "Neha Jain", saying this was her pre-marriage surname and brings proof in the form of a ration card/ passport/PAN card. What do you do?

7. You report a CT and the report is taken by the patient. Your colleague later shows you a renal calculus you missed. What do you do?

8. You report a CT and the report is taken by the patient. Your colleague later shows you a small subsegmental pulmonary embolus you missed. What do you do?

9. A patient with cancer comes for a follow-up CT. He says he forgot his previous CT at home, but says he needs the report urgently to show his doctor. What do you do?

10. A patient has taken away the films without a report. He calls for the report. What do you do? Do you issue a report based on the soft copy? Or do you insist on the films being deposited back?

Reports

A medical report, specifically a radiology report, is a medico-legal document, notwithstanding the "not for medicolegal use" that some centres and hospitals print behind or in the footer.

Hence, it is important to follow a set of standard rules related to reports.

1. A report cannot be changed or altered, once it is signed off and handed over to the patient. Many software systems do not allow alterations once signed off, while some allow changes to be made before the report is handed over to the patient or emailed. In any case, once the report is handed over to the patient, no change should be made.

2. If there is a discrepancy or a clarification needed, that has to be done in the form of an addendum. Even getting the age or the sex of the patient wrong needs to be addressed as an addendum and not by issuing a fresh report.

3. One major reason for this is that there is no guarantee that the patient will not have copied or photographed the report given initially. Giving a fresh, altered report, would in essence lead to a second copy of the report in circulation, which can become a medicolegal nightmare.

4. As far as possible, do not enter the clinical details in the report, unless you are absolutely sure, e.g. headache for 3 months, is vague and can be challenged by the patient and in turn lead to "headaches" for the radiologist and the centre/hospital concerned.

Answers

1. No and No. Issue an addendum.
2. Issue an addendum.
3. Issue an addendum.
4. Say no. Just don't do it.
5. Say no. You can't change a report already issued.
6. Reconfirm the finding. Issue an addendum with the new name. Keep a copy of the name change proof.
7. Issue an addendum report and proactively call the patient and inform the patient. This will prevent a future medicolegal issue of a "missed calculus".
8. Same answer as 7.
9. Issue a fresh report and when he comes back later with the old films, give an addendum with the comparison report. It is extra work, but can't be helped at times.
10. This depends on the centre's policy.

Chapter 10

The Radiologist and the Atomic Energy Regulation Board

Samir Gandhi

As per the Rules and Regulations framed by the Atomic Energy Regulation Board (AERB), each and every diagnostic X-ray producing unit like a routine radiographic machine, dental unit, OPG, mammography, CT scan, etc. is required to be registered with AERB. A center providing these facilities or possessing these machines also needs to be registered.

Following are the basic requirements to possess the above-mentioned pieces of equipment

1. Registration of the premises
2. Registration of the equipment
3. Registration of the radiation safety officer (RSO)
4. Monitoring of the persons exposed to radiation
5. Periodical quality assessment of the machines
6. Periodical renewal of the registration
7. Follow the rules prescribed by the AERB to minimize radiation hazards to clinic personnel, patients and environment.

The one nodal site which each radiologist must regularly visit for managing the processes related to AERB and the use of X-ray producing equipment is eLORA (e-Licensing of Radiation Application System) at https://elora.aerb.gov.in/ELORA/populateLoginAction.htm (there is no space bar anywhere despite the capital letters coming in between). All the pieces of information related to various AERB regulations are provided here.

Site Selection and Planning

Before the start of the radiology center, proper planning is required for placement of various pieces of equipment in the premises. The relevant guidelines and specific requirements are prescribed by AERB. Important ones include the size of the room, wall thickness, lead/radiation shielding, use of lead glass, etc.

A specific requirement which is a big hindrance for space crunched city dwellings is the prohibition of the use of two or more machines in the same room. Thus, a mammography unit, an OPG unit and a routine X-ray machine should be located in different rooms. Given the high real estate prices and increasing capital cost, this requirement has serious repercussions. The IRIA and other bodies have been pushing the AERB for alternative solutions such as using a 2-way switch, so that only 1 machine gets electric supply at any point of time.

Selection of Vendor and Machines

The eLORA site provides a detailed list of authorized vendors and machines, which is regularly updated. Before placing an order, especially for a lesser known machine or from a less known vendor, everyone should check their credentials on the eLORA site. Always demand up-to-date machine and vendor approval certificates issued by the AERB. Check for the approval of the specific model and make of the machine.

Registration of the Clinic and Machines and Renewals

A place intended to be used for installing X-ray generating equipment needs to be registered with AERB. The entire registration process is online, although it may prove to be a bit tedious and complicated. Similarly, all the machines that will be installed or are installed need to be registered as well.

The person responsible for implementation of the AERB guidelines, rules and regulations is designated the RSO (Radiation Safety Officer). In most cases, the radiologist or owner becomes the RSO. If the radiologist is not the owner and is merely reporting the radiographs, some other person who can meet the requirements should be appointed as the RSO.

The registration certificate should be displayed prominently in the clinic. The registration of the clinic has to be renewed every 5 years.

There are many agencies who provide services for facilitating registration. Any of these can be safely selected, provided they are registered and approved by the AERB. Check the eLORA site for the same. The charges may vary depending on the city, number of units to be registered, etc. It would be useful to look at more than one option and bargain hard. Try to fix a contract for regular QA services and renewal services as well. Be sure to take all the assurances and scope of work from the agency in writing.

One of the problems faced while registration is proof of business address. Documents accepted are:

1. Shop and establishment certificate (doctor's clinics are however now exempted from registration under Shop and Establishment Act).
2. PAN/TAN in clinic's name: Unfortunately, it is a common practice that being an ownership business entity, the PAN/TAN number is in the doctor's name and not in the clinic's name).
3. PCPNDT Registration Certificate: However, many facilities such as an orthopedic set-up or a dentist may not be registered under the PCPNDT Act.
4. Letter from the local corporator.

The IRIA and other bodies have suggested that a Notarized Declaration should be taken as proof of address along with the society's maintenance bill, a letter from the society, or a Leave and License Agreement Copy.

The requirement of a qualified technician may also often get difficult to fulfil. It is not easy to get an X-ray technician who is qualified as per AERB guidelines, particularly in tier-II and tier-III cities. There are many institutions who give training and certificates of qualification to X-ray technicians to individuals. Unfortunately, in real life, the degrees so awarded are often dubious and the knowledge of the candidate is substandard. There is no regulation in place to control teaching standards of these institutions. The IRIA and other bodies have suggested that the work experience of the person should be accepted as eligibility for becoming a qualified X-ray technician.

During the course of the eLORA registration, it is important to provide your personal email address and make sure that another person from the agency/center does not give his or her email address. All the relevant notices and information are going to be sent on the registered email address, and it is imperative to have your own email registered with AERB.

Monitoring of Persons Exposed to Radiation

All the persons who intend to use the X-ray generating equipment or who are exposed to radiation have to be registered with the AERB, and need to be issued thermoluminescent dosimeter (TLD) badges. This list includes not just the X-ray technician, but also members of the staff who regularly remain present in the X-ray room during exposure, such as nurses and assistants. Once a person is registered, his or her registration becomes permanent. If he or she resigns and joins another center, his/her registration number is transferred to the new center so that the radiation exposure history is continuously monitored.

There are specific guidelines regarding the use of the TLD badges, which everyone should be well versed with. The badge should be placed on the body as directed. When not in use, it should be kept out of the radiation producing room in a safe place.

The TLD badges are replaced every 3 months for exposure assessment. The dosimetry readings are provided for the last badge as also the cumulative dose. Any deviation from the normal range is immediately notified.

Periodic Quality Assurance Checks

It is mandatory to obtain a quality assurance (QA) report of each machine every 2 years. This is a relatively simple process. The QA agencies send their engineers with the necessary equipment. They evaluate the radiation emission from the machines, and the level of scattered radiation inside and outside the room. In the end, a report is provided and corrective measures advised if necessary. It is important to comply with the advice properly. The QA report should be filed regularly and should be easily available during inspection. The clinic staff and the radiographer should be aware of where it has been kept.

FEW DO'S

1. Follow the rules and guidelines as prescribed by the AERB. They are simple and uniform. Importantly, unlike the PCPNDT Act, there is no presumption of guilt.

2. Try to minimize radiation exposure to the staff, patients and environment as much as possible. Use lead aprons, lead glasses and gloves as and when necessary.

3. Put notices prominently in your clinic regarding precautions and guidelines about radiation. Display educational material for the benefit of the patients and their attendants. Such display cards are available at the eLORA website. Download and print them (example below; available online at the eLORA website, accessed on 25.7.2017).

4. Register your place and machines.

5. Get QA done every 2 years.

6. Renew your registration every 5 years.

7. Register all your staff who are exposed to radiations.

8. Inform changes in your staff to the TLD service provider.

9. If you are shifting or relocating, get the registration updated or get a new registration.

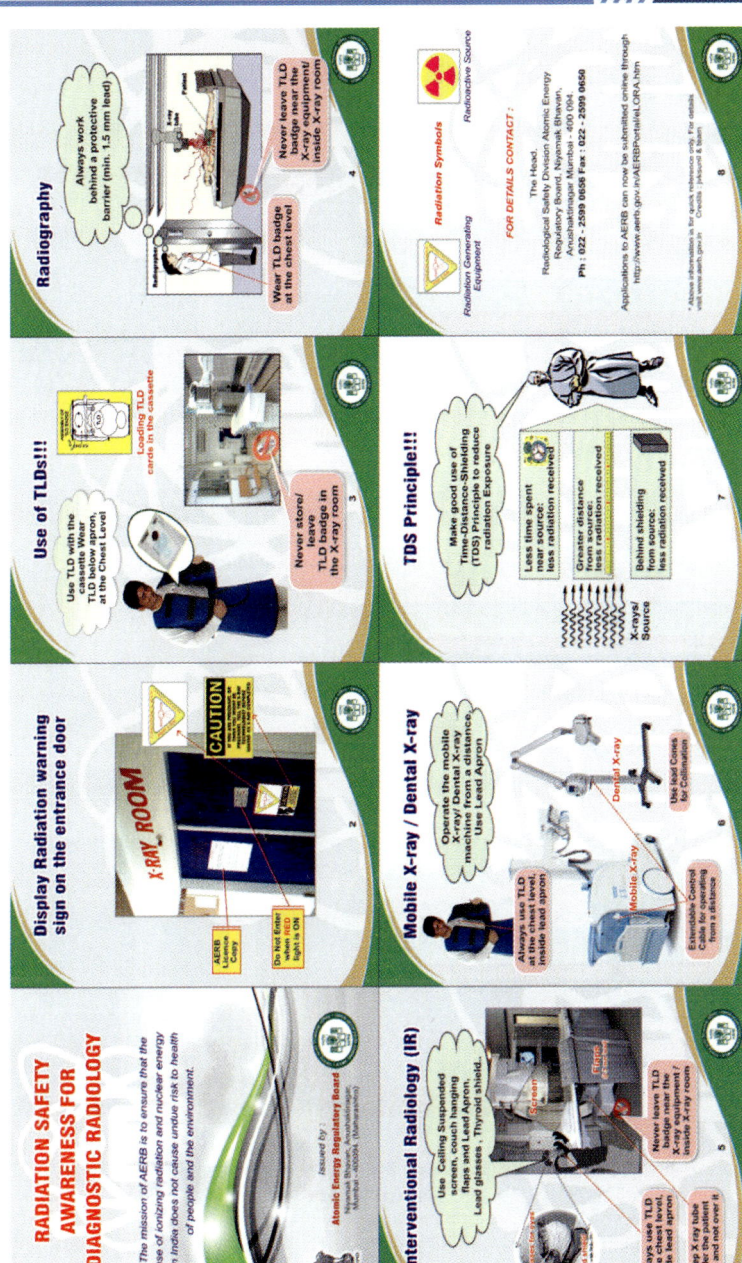

Radiation Safety in Fluoroscopy Procedures

■ Ways to Reduce of Radiation Dose to Staff and Patients

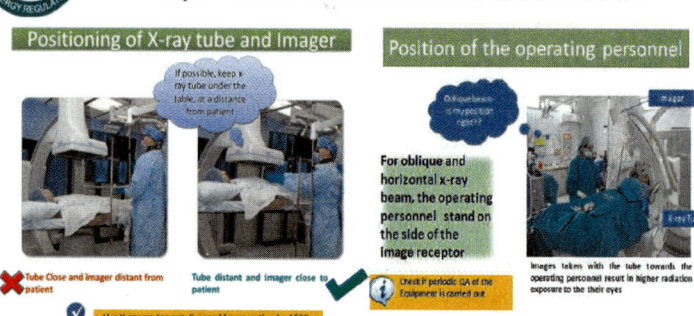

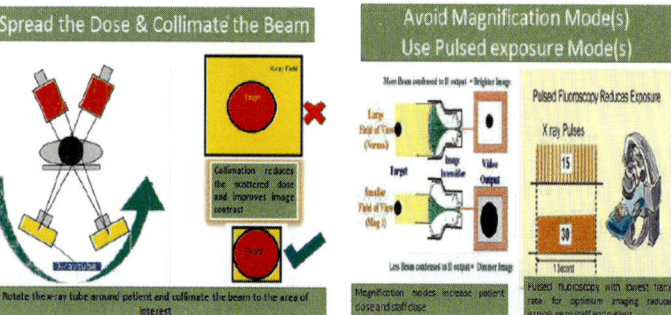

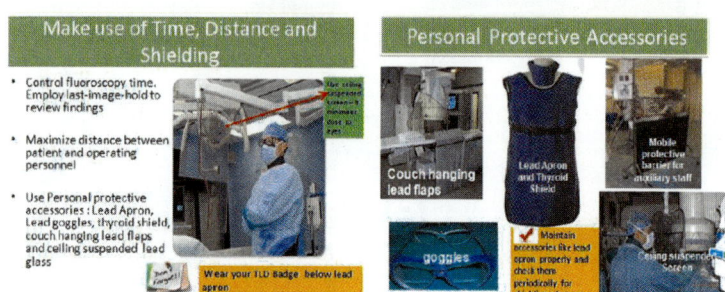

Issued By : Atomic Energy Regulatory Board, Niyamak Bhavan, Anushakti Nagar
Mumbai 400 094

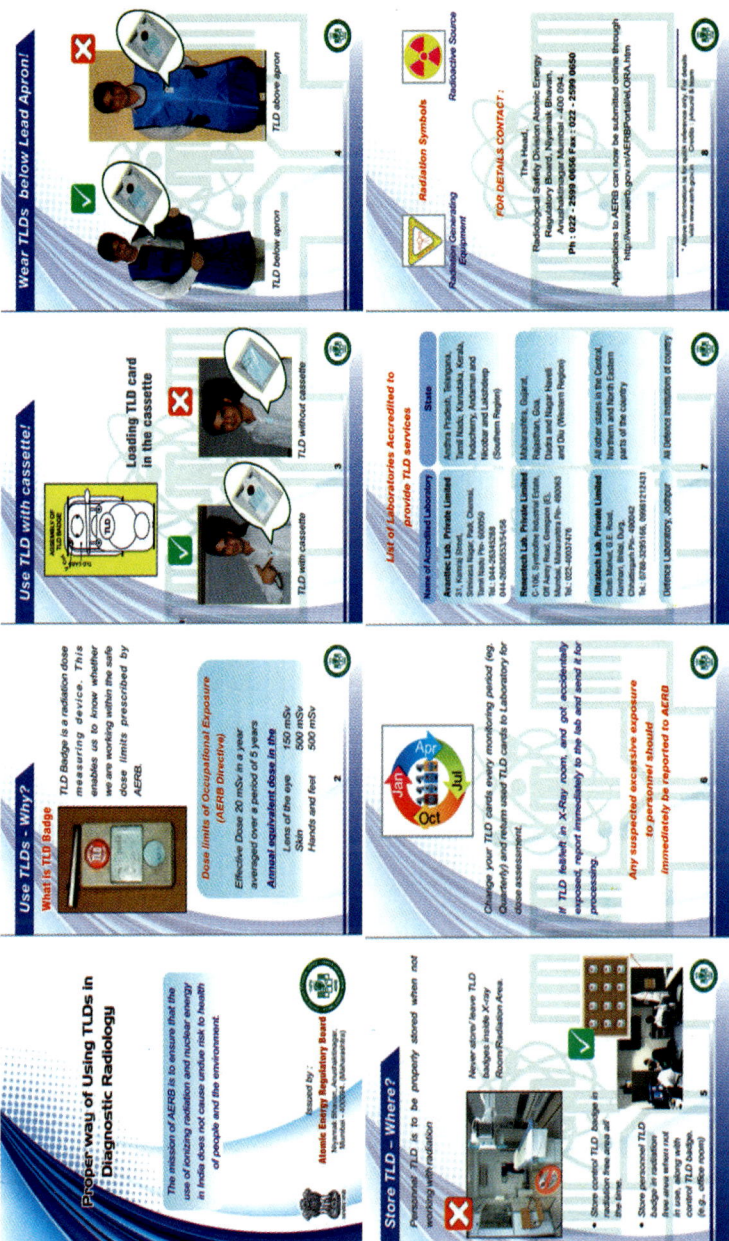

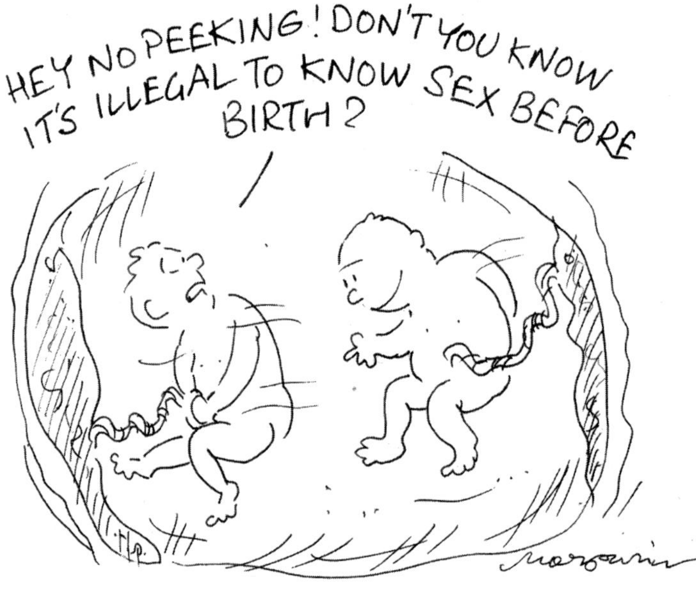
HEY NO PEEKING! DON'T YOU KNOW IT'S ILLEGAL TO KNOW SEX BEFORE BIRTH?

Chapter 11

Practical Pre-Conception Pre-Natal Sex Determination Act

Milind Gune

DISCLAIMER

This brief chapter is not an exhaustive discussion on the Pre-Conception Pre-Natal Sex Determination (PCPNDT) compliance issue. Rather; it is a practical listing of do's and don'ts for the radiology practitioner based on an important document circulated to the IRIA (Maharashtra State Branch of IRIA, Mumbai), amongst others, by the Rajya Kutumb Kalyan Karyalay, Pune, dated 04/08/2015 in reference to a decision taken by the Maharashtra State supervisory board on 17/06/2015.

As such, a few of these guidelines are Maharashtra state specific. However, these guidelines do distill the important points that the radiologist needs to know in his or her everyday practice.

The reader is encouraged to refer to his/her State Appropriate Authority (AA)/State branch of IRIA for state-specific practice guidelines. For example, the online form F submission and machine registration number are steps followed in Maharashtra and as such may not be applicable in other states. Please note that it is also likely that do's and don'ts applicable across India may soon be formulated. Please also read the section regarding references at the end of this chapter.

DO'S AND DON'TS FOR THE RADIOLOGIST PERFORMING ULTRASOUND EXAMINATIONS

Do's

1. Get registered with the concerned Appropriate Authority.
2. Apply in prescribed form A of the PCPNDT Act.
3. Attach all required documents like affidavit, undertaking degree, training certificate, registration with appropriate state medical board (MMC for Maharashtra), place details, equipment details and a cheque of the registration fees.
4. Do display certificate of registration form B of PCPNDT Act [one or two, original or xerox not specified in Act].
5. Apply for renewal at least one month prior to expiry of registration.
6. Carry out procedures only by the doctor whose name is written in form B.
7. Attach annexed list of doctors certified by AA, if no space on form B.
8. Conduct procedures only at approved place.
9. Use only equipment that is mentioned in form B.
10. Get the machine registration (MRC) number for the machine from the AA.
11. Inform any change in place, person or equipment at least one month before the AA and get it endorsed. (Delhi High Court directed for the time period to be one week.)
12. Keep at least one copy of the PCPNDT Act at the centre. Please do check with your state AA/local IRIA chapter regarding this guideline.
13. Display the timings of the doctor performing procedures at the place of work.
14. Obtain written declaration of pregnant women on "F" form and preserve it. (New 'F' form having ABCD parts).
15. Maintain register as per Rule 9(1).
16. Take a printout of online "F" form, authenticated by the doctor performing the procedure. The patient need not

wait for signing the declaration on printout copy. Hard copy of any one to be preserved.

17. Send monthly report by 5th day of the following month.

18. Preserve the records for 2 years. If any case is going on in court, then preserve them till the case is disposed of.

19. Display board in English and Marathi (or appropriate local language) "Disclosure of the sex of the fetus is prohibited under law".

20. Surrender certificate of registration if there is change in ownership (as certificate is non-transferable).

21. Apply for fresh registration if there is change in ownership (as certificate is non-transferable).

22. Write name and designation of the person performing the procedure under his/her signature, and the date of the procedure.

23. Keep all records as:
    - D, E or F forms as applicable.
    - G form (if invasive procedure).
    - Sonography plates.
    - Referral slips (details if self-referral).

24. Do provide records for inspection to the AA or person authorized.

25. Ask for a copy of the inspection report from the AA after the inspection is over.

26. Do make an appeal to the State AA under Rule 19(2), if aggrieved by the decision of the District/Corporation AA.

Don'ts

1. Don't conduct sonography without a referral slip, clearly stating the reason for the sonography.

2. Don't communicate sex of the fetus by any manner or sign, verbal or otherwise.

3. Don't purchase machine without intimating the AA.

4. Don't change place without intimating the AA.

5. Don't employ or cause to be employed any non-qualified person to conduct the sonography.

6. Don't change any sonologist without intimating the local AA and getting the name added/deleted in form B.

7. Don't publish any advertisement in any form for pre-natal determination of fetal sex.

8. Don't transfer certificate of registration to any person, organization or company.

While the above is not an exhaustive list of the guidelines, it does form a template for each local IRIA chapter to inform its members regarding local standard operating procedures/guidelines in collaboration with their local AA.

BIBLIOGRAPHY

1. http://pcpndt.raj.nic.in/
2. https://pcpndt.maharashtra.gov.in/Home/Login.aspx
3. The PC-PNCDT Act itself-http://rajswasthya. nic.in/PCPNDT% 2005.12.08/PCPNDT% 20Act%20(2).pdf

Glossary

NCRP: National Council on Radiation Protection and Measurements

ICRP: International Council on Radiation Protection

ACR: American College of Radiology

CECT: Contrast-enhanced CT

CE-MRI: Contrast-enhanced MRI

ESUR: European Society of Urogenital Radiology

US-FDA: US Food and Drug Administration

IRIA: Indian Radiological and Imaging Association

AERB: Atomic Energy Regulation Board

PCPNDT Act: Pre-Conception Pre-Natal Sex Determination Act